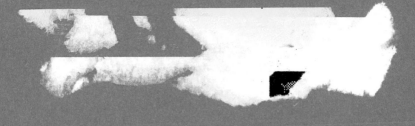

THE TEAR FILM

Publisher: Caroline Makepeace
Development editor: Robert Edwards
Production Controller: Chris Jarvis
Desk editor: Claire Hutchins
Cover designer: Alan Studholme

THE TEAR FILM:
structure, function and clinical examination

Donald R. Korb, Jennifer Craig,
Michael Doughty, Jean-Pierre Guillon,
George Smith and Alan Tomlinson

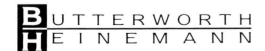

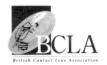

OXFORD   AMSTERDAM   BOSTON   LONDON   NEW YORK
SAN DIEGO   SAN FRANCISCO   SINGAPORE   SYDNEY

Butterworth-Heinemann
An imprint of Elsevier Science

First published 2002

ISBN 0 7506 4196 7

British Library Cataloguing in Publication Data
A catalogue record for this book is available from the
British Library

Library of Congress Cataloguing in Publication Data
A catalog record for this book is available from the
Library of Congress

612.841
b00781

Composition by Genesis Typesetting, Laser Quay, Rochester, Kent
Printed and bound in Italy

II

Contents List

Introduction: the importance of the tear film

In the evolutionary journey from aquatic-based life forms to land-dwelling organisms, a significant anatomical feature developed within the ocular system to prevent the desiccation of the anterior segment. This 'lacrimal system', in conjunction with other accessory glands and blinking mechanisms, allowed the integrity of the epithelial surfaces of the globe and conjunctiva to be maintained in a terrestrial environment. This system remains critically important for ocular health and function today.

The importance of tears has long been recognized. In the fifth to fourth centuries BC, Hippocrates classified ophthalmic conditions as dry or humid (Murube, 1992). In 1946, Wolff presented the concept of a three-layered tear film structure – the mucin layer, the aqueous layer, and the lipid layer – which has become the universally accepted model. The nature of these three layers has received increasing attention over the past 50 years and the present acceleration of knowledge in all areas of the tear film is the primary reason for this text.

To appreciate the importance of the tear film, it is instructive to examine the consequences of compromised tear film and 'dry eye disorders', which can range from the commonly reported symptoms of soreness and scratchiness (McMonnies and Ho, 1986) to the more severe conditions of ocular surface damage, decreased vision (Lemp, 1995), and contact lens intolerance (Korb and Henriquez, 1980). Furthermore, the very high prevalence of dry eye symptoms, reportedly 10–25 per cent of the general adult population (Bandeen-Roche et al., 1997; Doughty et al., 1997; Schein et al., 1997) and 18–30 per cent of soft contact lens wearers (Orsborn and Zantos, 1989), emphasizes the importance of the tear film in clinical practice. It appears that the tear film impacts the contact lens practitioner more than any other eye practitioner, with the exception of those in specialty dry eye practices. The reason is that the majority of contact lens problems, including intolerance and limited wearing time, are tear film related. These difficulties are caused by the physical disruption and increased evaporation of the tear film caused by the contact lens, especially when the tear film is marginal without the presence of a contact lens (Hathaway and Lowther, 1978; Brennan and Efron, 1989; Orsborn and Roddy, 1989; Bandeen-Roche et al., 1997).

The relevant question for the clinician is whether the large volume of information about the tear film, generated by rapid technological advances, can be translated into a greater understanding of and capability for the diagnosis and treatment of dry eye disorders. Complicating this question is the lack of standardized definitions for the terminology of tear film-related disorders. The National Eye Institute addressed this issue of standardization by sponsoring a workshop on Clinical Trials in Dry Eyes in 1993–1994 (Lemp, 1995). A 'global definition' of dry eye was presented as follows:

> Dry eye is a disorder of the tear film due to tear deficiency or excessive tear evaporation which causes damage to the inter-palpebral ocular surface and is associated with symptoms of ocular discomfort.

This definition was put forward with an expressed recognition of its limitations and that it does not attribute dry eye disorders to specific causes. The workshop members also defined a set of global criteria and applicable tests for dry eye, and established that most forms of dry eye would exhibit the following features:

1. Symptoms, as demonstrated by a validated questionnaire
2. Interpalpebral surface damage
3. Tear instability
4. Tear hyperosmolarity.

Again, it is important to stress that these are minimum operating guidelines for the assessment of dry eye conditions and may need to be modified based upon individual situations.

The often enigmatic nature of dry eye syndrome requires the clinician to customize his diagnostic approach and treatment regimen for the individual patient, as symptoms do not always correlate with signs and vice versa. This dichotomy is particularly relevant with regard to contact lens wearers; in fact, recognition of the contact lens-induced dry eye (Tomlinson, 1992) and the 'questionably or marginally dry eye' patient (Mackie and Seal, 1981; Nilsson and Anderson, 1986) has been a significant driving force underlying recent research. The understanding that lifestyle and environmental factors, such as plane travel (Rocher and Fatt, 1995), visual display terminals (Patel et al., 1991; Sheedy, 1993; Tsubota and Nakamori, 1993), seasonal or climatic changes (Fatt and Rocher, 1994), indoor climates (Franck, 1986), air turbulence (Rolando and Refojo, 1983), or 'sick building syndrome' (Franck, 1991), can provoke dry eye complaints, emphasizes the important role of the patient questionnaire in obtaining the information necessary to understand the aetiology of the underlying disorder.

Evaluation of the tear film is both established and evolving. Mathers *et al.* (1996) have succinctly summarized contemporary tear film evaluation as follows:

> There is as yet no single test that completely evaluates the ocular tear film. Each test alone examines part of the process but does not explain the entire process sufficiently. It is only when these tests are seen together that we get a more complete look at this dynamic process.

The goal of this text is to provide a comprehensive review and understanding of the tear film, its evaluation and its treatment, in light of recent research. Emphasis is placed on those aspects that are of relevance to both primary eye care and contact lens practice, including:

- The surface features of the cornea and conjunctiva, including how their design and function supports the tear film, discussed by Professor Michael Doughty, whose expertise as a scientist specializing in these areas provides a unique insight and a helpful summary for the clinician.
- A comprehensive overview of the tear film structure and function, presented by Dr Jennifer Craig, including relevant secretory mechanisms, related anatomy, and the relationship between the tear film and contact lens wear.
- The clinical techniques available for the study of the tear film and its components, reviewed by Dr Jean-Pierre Guillon. This information is particularly valuable for distinguishing between the various types of dry eye that present in the clinical setting. Diagnostic methods for the differentiation of the normal from the compromised tear film, including new methods of evaluation of the lipid layer are presented.
- Age-related changes of the tear film, discussed in depth by Professor Alan Tomlinson, including the question of whether dry eye is an inevitable consequence of the normal ageing process. The potential influence of genetic and environmental factors and the capacity of the tear film system to compensate for age-related changes in its physiology are reviewed.
- The pathology of the tear film and the more common manifestations of such abnormalities observed in the clinical setting, presented by Mr George Smith, whose expertise as a consultant ophthalmologist brings insight and strategies for the diagnosis and treatment of dry eye disorders.
- Current and new concepts for the evaluation of tear film stability, ocular surface staining, new concepts in the examination of the lipid

layer, and a strategy in sequence of testing for the tear film, discussed by Dr Donald Korb. Also included are the results of a survey of 68 ophthalmologists and optometrists with recognized expertise in dry eye disorders concerning their choices of diagnostic tests.

It is hoped that this information will provide a review of contemporary knowledge, encourage differential diagnosis of tear film disorders, and improve the management and treatment of the dry eye patient.

References

Bandeen-Roche, K., Munoz, B., Tielsch, J. M. *et al.* (1997) Self-reported assessment of dry eye in a population-based setting. *Invest. Ophthalmol. Vis. Sci.*, **38,** 2469–2475.

Brennan, N. A. and Efron, N. (1989) Symptomatology of HEMA contact lens wear. *Optom. Vis. Sci.*, **66,** 834–838.

Doughty, M. J., Fonn, D., Richter, D. *et al.* (1997) A patient questionnaire approach to estimating the prevalence of dry eye symptoms in patients presenting to optometric practices across Canada. *Optom. Vis. Sci.*, **74,** 624–631.

Fatt, I. and Rocher, P. (1994) Contact lens performance in different climates. *Optom. Today,* **34,** 26.

Franck, C. (1986) Eye symptoms and signs in buildings with indoor climate problems. *Acta Ophthalmol.*, **64,** 306.

Franck, C. (1991) Fatty layer of the precorneal tear film in the 'office eye syndrome'. *Acta Ophthalmol.*, **69,** 737–743.

Hathaway, R. A. and Lowther, G. E. (1978) Factors influencing the rate of deposit formation on hydrophilic lenses. *Aust. J. Optom.*, **61,** 92.

Korb, D. R. and Henriquez, A. S. (1980) Meibomian gland dysfunction and contact lens intolerance. *J. Am. Optom. Assoc.*, **51,** 243–251.

Lemp, M. A. (1995) Report of the National Eye Institute/Industry Workshop on Clinical Trials in Dry Eyes. *CLAO J.*, **21,** 221–232.

Mackie, I. A. and Seal, D. V. (1981) The questionably dry eye. *Br. J. Ophthalmol.*, **65,** 2–9.

Mathers, W. D., Lane, J. A. and Zimmerman, M. B. (1996) Tear film changes associated with normal aging. *Cornea*, **15,** 229.

McMonnies, C. W. and Ho, A. (1986) Marginal dry eye diagnosis: history versus biomicroscopy. In *The Preocular Tear Film in Health, Disease, and Contact Lens Wear* (ed. F. J. Holly), Lubbock, Dry Eye Institute, pp. 32–40.

Murube, J. (1992) Hippocratium Corpus. In *The Dry Eye. A Comprehensive Guide* (eds M. A. Lemp and R. Marquardt), Berlin, Springer-Verlag, p. 5.

Nilsson, S. E. G. and Anderson, L. (1986) Contact lens wear in dry environments. *Acta Ophthalmol.*, **64,** 221–225.

Orsborn, G. N. and Roddy, M. (1989) Hydrogel lenses and dry eye symptoms. *J. Br. Cont. Lens Assoc.*, **6,** 37.

Orsborn, G. N. and Zantos, S. G. (1989) Practitioner survey: management of dry-eye symptoms in soft lens wearers. *Cont. Lens Spectrum*, **4**, 23–26.

Patel, S., Henderson, R., Bradley, L. *et al.* (1991) Effect of visual display unit use on blink rate and tear stability. *Optom. Vis. Sci.*, **68**, 888.

Rocher, P. and Fatt, I. (1995) Hydrogel contact lenses: air temperature and relative humidity in man-made environments which may influence evaporation from a hydrogel contact lens on the eye. *Optom. Today*, **35**, 22.

Rolando, M. and Refojo, M. F. (1983) Tear evaporimeter for measuring water evaporation rate from the tear film under controlled conditions in humans. *Exp. Eye Res.*, **36**, 25–33.

Schein, O. D., Munoz, B., Tielsch, J. M. *et al.* (1997) Prevalence of dry eye among the elderly. *Am. J. Ophthalmol.*, **124**, 723–728.

Sheedy, J. E. (1993) Dry eye at VDTs. *Eyecare Technol.*, **6**, 52–79.

Tomlinson, A. (1992) Contact lens-induced dry eye. In *Complications of Contact Lens Wear* (ed. A. Tomlinson), St Louis, Mosby, pp. 195–218.

Tsubota, K. and Nakamori, K. (1993) Dry eyes and video display terminals. Letter to the Editor. *N. Engl. J. Med.*, **328**, 524.

Wolff, E. (1946) The muco-cutaneous junction of the lid margin and the distribution of tear fluid. *Trans. Ophthalmol. Soc.*, **66**, 291–308.

Authors

Chapter 1: The cornea and conjunctival surfaces in relation to the tear film
Michael Doughty is a Research Professor in the Department of Vision Sciences at Glasgow Caledonian University, Glasgow, UK

Chapter 2: Structure and function of the preocular tear film
Chapter 4: Time and the tear film
Jennifer Craig is the Desmond Hadden Lecturer in Ophthalmology at the University of Auckland, New Zealand

Chapter 3: Current clinical techniques to study the tear film and tear secretions
Jean-Pierre Guillon works at the Centre for Ophthalmology and Visual Science Lions eye Institute, Nedlands, Western Australia

Chapter 4: Time and the tear film
Alan Tomlinson is Professor and Head of the Department of Vision Sciences, Glasgow Caledonian University, Glasgow, UK

Chapter 5: Pathology of the tear film
George Smith is Consultant Ophthalmic Surgeon and Director of Corneal Services at Coventry and Warwickshire Hospital, Coventry, UK

Chapter 6: The tear film – its role today and in the future
Donald R. Korb is Clinical Professor at the School of Optometry, Berkeley and Director of Research at Ocular Research of Boston, Boston, USA

1 The cornea and conjunctival surfaces in relation to the tear film

Michael Doughty

Introduction

Basic organization of the conjunctival and corneal surfaces

The tear film is often referred to as the 'pre-corneal tear film' because this aspect is so easily evaluated. However, the tear film is in contact with a much larger ocular surface. The tear meniscus is obviously in contact with the bulbar conjunctiva and the eyelid margin and this should serve as a reminder that the tear film is also in contact with the rest of the conjunctiva.

Gross descriptive anatomy of the ocular surface

Based on whole eye histological examinations, it is possible to divide the ocular surface into eight zones as follows:

1. Corneal epithelium
2. Limbal epithelium
3. Bulbar conjunctival epithelium
4. Fornix conjunctival surfaces (upper and lower)
5. Orbital conjunctival surfaces (upper and lower)
6. Tarsal conjunctiva (principally upper)
7. Marginal conjunctival surfaces (upper and lower)
8. Muco-cutaneous edge of eyelids (upper and lower).

General descriptions and quantitative analyses of the human ocular surface anatomy need to consider the ethnic origins of the individuals concerned and a detailed review is beyond the scope of this chapter. However, in general terms, the normal human cornea has a horizontal diameter of between 9.5 and 13.5 mm. Smaller values would be expected in new-borns and infants but it is generally considered that a stable value is reached by 2–3 years of age (Smith, 1890; Hymes, 1929), after which little further change occurs. The horizontal palpebral aperture also shows an early age-dependence, with the full-sized aperture usually evident by early teens (Hymes, 1929). Such developmental changes are likely to differ between ethnic groups, most notably when comparing Caucasian with Oriental eyes. For Caucasians, the average vertical palpebral aperture can be expected to be between 7.5 and 11.5 mm, the smaller values being found in older individuals (Fox, 1966; Bruckner *et al.*, 1987; Fonn *et al.*, 1996; Zaman *et al.*, 1998).

The surface area of the adult (Caucasian) human cornea has been reported to be close to 1 cm^2 (Watsky *et al.*, 1988). The actual exposed ocular surface that includes the bulbar conjunctiva is dependent on the vertical palpebral aperture, and also depends on the mathematical formulae used to calculate the curved surface and its area (Rolando and Refojo, 1983; Sotayama *et al.*, 1995; Tiffany *et al.*, 1998; Zaman *et al.*, 1998). A reasonable estimate of the exposed ocular surface would be between 1.25 and 1.75 cm^2, depending on the habitual position of the upper eyelid, which can be influenced by the direction of gaze. The rest of the ocular surface under the eyelids is much larger than the exposed surface and has been estimated at more than 10 times that of the corneal surface (Watsky *et al.*, 1988).

Light microscopic evaluation of ocular surface cells

The 'precorneal' tear film is presumed to cover and lubricate the entire ocular surface all the way to the mid-point of the mucocutaneous zone at the margin of the eyelids. The entire surface is composed of various types of epithelial cells. There has been relatively little systematic examination of the eight regions, either by high-magnification light microscopy or by electron microscopy, and, as a consequence, it is usual for rather general and non-specific descriptions to be used. The cells are, however, distinctly different at different locations across the ocular surface and can be characterized as follows:

- Squamous stratified epithelium of the cornea
- Stratified/columnar limbal epithelial cells
- Cuboidal bulbar conjunctival epithelial cells with goblet cells
- Cuboidal orbital conjunctival epithelial cells with goblet cells
- Stratified/columnar fornix epithelial cells with goblet cells
- Cuboidal/stratified tarsal epithelial cells with goblet cells
- Stratified/cuboidal marginal conjunctival epithelial cells
- Muco-cutaneous junction.

The central corneal epithelium in man is composed of five to seven layers of cells that are traditionally divided into three groups: the basal, intermediate (wing) and superficial (squamous) cells (Ehlers, 1970). The limbal epithelium is also composed of several layers of cells but the stratification is less obvious. The limbal cells also differ from those of the corneal epithelium in that the cell surfaces are covered with a unique group of glycoproteins (including the cytokeratins) that are not found on the corneal cells and vice versa (Lange *et al.*, 1989; Wei *et al.*, 1995; Wolosin and Wang, 1995). The origins of these different surface glycoproteins relate to lineage of these cells through the stem cells.

The epithelium of the bulbar conjunctiva is generally composed of simple cuboidal cells with no obvious stratification (Srinivastan *et al.*, 1977; Weyruach, 1983; Lange *et al.*, 1989; Lawrenson and Ruskell, 1991; Wolosin and Wang, 1995). These cells are essentially a supporting matrix for the very numerous goblet cells that are present. The fornix epithelium is principally composed of simple cuboidal cells through which course the outlet ducts from the accessory and main lacrimal glands (Weyrauch, 1983; Huang *et al.*, 1988; Goller and Weyrauch, 1993; Wei *et al.*, 1995). There are also very high numbers of goblet cells.

The orbital zone of the palpebral conjunctiva is composed of cuboidal cells (Weyrauch, 1983; Huang *et al.*, 1988; Goller and Weyrauch, 1993; Wei *et al.*, 1995) that also form a supporting matrix for large numbers of goblet cells. The tarsal zone of the palpebral conjunctiva is composed of cuboidal cells with some degree of stratification. A modest number of goblet cells are found across this part of the ocular surface. At the junction between the tarsal and orbital zones of the palpebral conjunctiva are the outlets of the tarsal accessory lacrimal glands.

The marginal conjunctival surface is composed of cells with a relatively high degree of stratification into basal and superficial cells. There is some evidence that there is a narrow band of squamous epithelium just behind the orifices of the meibomian glands (also known as the tarsal glands of Meibom) (Doughty, 1997; Doughty and Bergmanson, 1999). The ocular mucocutaneous epithelium is thicker still compared to the marginal palpebral conjunctiva and clearly developed into distinct layers of cells (Wolff, 1964; Doughty and Bergmanson, 1999).

Surface characteristics of the conjunctiva and cornea

Assessment of the cells of the ocular surface by histological techniques reveals few differences between the epithelia across different parts of the ocular surface, beyond the fact that the numbers of layers of cells and the type of layering can be variable. However, viewing the various parts of the ocular surface directly reveals several more differences.

Scanning electron microscopy of the ocular surfaces

Scanning electron microscopy (SEM) shows that the surface characteristics of different parts of the ocular surface are not the same and that a considerable range of features can be observed (Doughty, 1997; Table 1.1).

The corneal epithelium is a mosaic of heterogeneous cells, both with respect to their size and surface features. There is a substantial range of cell sizes, i.e. the exposed surface areas of the superficial cells range from very small indeed (c. $5\,\mu m^2$) to very large (up to $2500\,\mu m^2$) (Doughty, 1990). There are subtle size (cell surface area) differences between central and peripheral cornea (Doughty and Fong, 1992). Differences in the surface density of cell surface microplicae mean that the cells have three main types of appearance which, for want of a better classification, have become known as 'light', 'medium' and 'dark' cells (Doughty, 1990).

Various theories have been proposed to explain these differences (Doughty, 1996a). For example, the cells could have different appearances because, while initially all of one type (lineage), they have undergone different types of terminal changes. A common explanation found in the

Table 1.1 Comparison of the morphological features of the surface cells of the corneal epithelium and palpebral conjunctiva

	Peripheral corneal epithelium	*Bulbar conjunctiva*	*Orbital conjunctiva*	*Tarsal conjunctiva*
General appearance in scanning electron microscopy	Light, medium and dark	Light and medium	Medium	Light and dark
Squamous	Yes	No	No	Possibly
Character of surface features	Microplicae	Microplicae, few microvilli	Microvilli	Microplicae, few microvilli
Packing of surface features	Dense	Moderate to dense	Moderate	Moderate to very dense
Cell–cell borders	Often straight	Straight or rounded	Generally rounded	Straight or rounded
Cell–cell interface (border) detail	Uniform and well-defined caulking-like material	Poorly-defined caulking-like material	No caulking-like material evident	No caulking-like material evident

literature is that the dark cells represent those with the greatest terminal changes as a result of having been resident on the ocular surface for the longest period of time, i.e. several hours or up to a few days. In such a scheme, it is the dark cells that are more prone to desquamation (Begley *et al.*, 1998) and the light cells represent cells recently arrived at the ocular surface from the underlying layers. However, evidence has also been presented that 'light' cells can be shown to exfoliate and on this basis the different appearances of the cells has been proposed to be the result of them all being terminally differentiated cells from at least three different lineages (Doughty, 1996a).

The surface microplicae of the corneal epithelial cells can be present at different densities on the light, medium and dark cells. At extremely high magnification, the actual surface of the microplicae appears to be composed of rows of large bead-like molecules that could be the glycocalyx. The pristine corneal surface can be shown to be almost (> 99 per cent) intact, with distinct proportions of the three cell types (Doughty, 1990) and just a few desquamating (exfoliating) cells (the squamous cells). The squamous cells readily separate from the corneal surface (e.g. with saline irrigation) and human studies suggest that more cells are readily shed at the start and end of the day (Begley *et al.*, 1998). For rabbit cornea, the occasional application of a preservative-containing artificial tear, for example, can mildly increase desquamation (Doughty, 1992), although the epithelium appears to be able to adapt with continued use. However, with extended treatment with isotonic saline (Doughty, 1995), gross desquamation and surface cell alteration can develop. A mucous, aqueous or lipid layer would be most unlikely to form over such a surface of desquamating cells.

The limbal and bulbar conjunctival cells also have light and medium, and perhaps dark surface appearance characteristics, but squamous cells are uncommon and the overall size and range of cell sizes is very much smaller than that observed for the corneal epithelium (Doughty, Unpublished studies). A distinct transition can be seen between the peripheral corneal epithelium and the surrounding conjunctiva. The orbital conjunctiva has a remarkably different appearance in that the cells are homogeneous and have a medium appearance under SEM. The cells are relatively small and with cell surface areas only ranging from $20–200\,\mu m^2$ (average $75\,\mu m^2$) (Doughty, 1997). Squamous cells do not appear to be present.

The surface cells of the tarsal conjunctiva are, however, different again and have distinct light or dark appearances as a result of microplicae and microvilli on their surfaces (Doughty, 1997). The cells are relatively small and only a modest range of cell surface areas of $15–300\,\mu m^2$ (average $90\,\mu m^2$) has been found for the rabbit tarsal conjunctiva (Doughty, 1997). Squamous cells do not appear to be present.

A rather marked transition then occurs on the ocular surface at the marginal zone where the orifices of the meibomian glands are located. The cells surrounding the orifices lose their light and dark characteristics and appear to be squamous (Doughty, 1997). This is presumably a rather unique aspect of the oculo-mucocutaneous zone of the ocular surface and light microscopy and transmission electron microscopy (TEM) studies indicate that these desquamating cells form the most superficial aspect of a substantial stratified epithelium much thicker than that on the adjacent tarsal conjunctiva (Wolff, 1964; Doughty and Bergmanson, 1999).

Just beyond the oculo-mucocutaneous junction, and just proximal to the insertion of the eyelashes, is a zone covered with dead, desquamated cells (Doughty and Panju, 1995; Greiner et al., 1997). The relatively large size of the cells suggests that most originate from the corneal epithelium. Underlying this 'garbage zone' is a stratified epithelium with distinctive keratinization of the most superficial cells (Doughty and Bergmanson, 1999).

Impression cytology

Samples of cells taken by impression cytology can be graded as being normal through to metaplastic, with cells of a similar appearance obtained from bulbar and tarsal conjunctiva (Rivas et al., 1992). Grading is based on the relative area of the cells occupied by the nucleus compared to the surrounding cytoplasm. Normal cells have nucleus to cytoplasm ratios (N:C ratios) of 1:1 or 1:2 and values up to 1:8 being reported in conditions such as dry eye (Knop and Brewitt, 1992). Similar cells can be obtained from both the bulbar and tarsal conjunctiva (Rivas et al., 1992).

More recently, cells obtained by impression cytology have been subjected to quantitative analysis. Cells from the corneal surface (via a contact lens) are generally larger, and have dimensions and areas that are consistent with SEM morphometry, i.e. cell dimensions of 10–60 µm and cell surface areas of 75–1900 µm^2 (Laurent and Wilson, 1997). By morphometric analyses, these corneal cells are essentially indistinguishable from the range of bulbar conjunctival cells that can be collected from individuals with no overt ocular surface disease (Doughty et al., 2000), i.e. just because a cell is 'large' does not mean it is a corneal epithelial cell as opposed to a conjunctival cell (and vice versa).

Impression cytology, with morphometry, of what are considered 'normal' (healthy) human bulbar conjunctival cells reveals relatively homogeneous smaller cells with surface areas ranging from just 25–250 µm^2, with an average of just over 100 µm^2. However, following extended but mild irritation of the eye, these cells develop metaplastic characteristics with a significant (4×) enlargement of cell area and increase in the visually-estimated N:C ratios from <1:2 to around 1:6 (Blades *et al.*, 1998). Based on actual measures of cyoplasm and nucleus areas from cells collected by impression cytology, normal human bulbar conjunctival cells can be expected to have a grade 0 appearance and an N:C ratio between 0.983 and 0.531 (Blades and Doughty, 2000).

Biomicroscopy of the tarsal conjunctiva using fluorescein dye

The cells on the tarsal conjunctival surface appear to be divided up into larger discrete groups as evidenced by a reticular pattern visualized *in vivo* with fluorescein dye). These domains can be assessed by morphometry and have much larger areas than cells, with average values around $45\,000\,\mu m^2$, and a range of 5000 to almost $25\,000\,\mu m^2$ (Potvin *et al.*, 1994; Doughty *et al.*, 1995). Based on morphometry assessments, it appears that these zones can coalescence when some inflammatory conditions develop, e.g. in contact lens-associated papillary conjunctivitis, where domain areas may be more than $1\,mm^2$ (Doughty *et al.*, 1995).

Interaction of dyes and stains with the ocular surface and tear film

The reason for the fluorescein-visualized reticular pattern on the tarsal conjunctiva is unknown and it develops without any special measures being taken. Since a similar pattern can develop on the corneal surface after instillation of fluorescein and gentle rubbing of the eyelids against the cornea, the fluorescein could be forming an imprint on the corneal surface and off the tarsal conjunctiva. Alternatively, the corneal surface may be similarly organized into discrete zones.

Such uncertainty arises because it is still not understood how fluorescein interacts with the ocular surface. Fluorescein can reveal minute zones of hyperfluorescence that have traditionally been considered to reflect portions of disrupted epithelial cells, e.g. 3 and 9 o'clock staining patterns or a superficial punctate keratopathy (Wilson *et al.*, 1995), although the dye can permeate some, presumably compromised cells. The size of such discrete zones of hyperfluorescence would suggest that they include small numbers of cells (Wilson *et al.*, 1995) that are damaged or at least resistant to being covered by mucus (Bitton and Lovasik, 1998). When fluorescein is added to the tear film, a uniform fluorescein film can be seen briefly after which tear 'break-up' occurs and darker regions develop in the film. The shape and kinetics of these hypofluorescent patterns have been quantified (Bitton and Lovasik, 1998), and also indicates that only discrete groups of cells are involved when the tear film is unstable.

Contemporary research on fluorescein and rose bengal suggests that the hyperfluorescent patterns visualized on the corneal surface are not simply due to damaged cells. Rose bengal has traditionally been considered to be a 'vital' stain in that it will impart a (crimson) coloration to devitalized cells (Doughty, 1996b). Recent studies however suggest that such staining will occur for cells that are deficient in their surface mucous coat, i.e. the normal glycocalyx and/or its mucous covering on the cell surfaces blocks rose bengal penetration into the cells (Tseng and Zhang, 1995). It is possible that aspects of fluorescein dye interaction with ocular surface cells may also be dependent on the characteristics of the overlying glycocalyx and/or tear film biophysics. Lastly, recent evidence suggests that fluorescein can migrate from one corneal surface cell to an adjacent one and that such inter-cellular transfer reflects cell–cell communication via gap junctions (Williams and Watsky, 1996). What is perhaps most interesting is that the transfer of a fluorescein derivative (carboxyfluorescein) can also occur between cells immediately below the superficial cells. The vitality of the gap junctions is considered to be an indicator of the 'health' of the cell layer.

Underlying features of the conjunctiva and cornea

The cells across the ocular surface cells have a range of characteristics and this may be partly due to the fact that there are a range of underlying features, some of which are directly in communication with the ocular surfaces.

Transmission electron microscopy of epithelial cells, secretory cells and secretory organs of the ocular surface

A feature of most if not all of normal epithelial cells of the ocular surface is that transmission electron microscopy (TEM) shows the cell surfaces to be formed into very small projections (Takakusaki, 1969; Rohen and Steuhl, 1982; Nichols, 1996). TEM cannot distinguish between these being individual spikes on the surface of the cells (i.e. microvilli) or to be sections through micro-undulations of the cell surfaces (i.e. microplicae). Different parts of the ocular surface have microplicae or microvilli, and sometimes both.

TEM also shows the superficial (squamous) cells of the corneal epithelium to be very attenuated in thickness, yet should be tightly connected together via a series of cell–cell junctions called zonula occludens (Sugrue and Zieske, 1997), and these are perhaps related to the 'caulking-like substance' seen along the cell–cell borders in SEM. Slightly deeper lying cells are linked by an immature form of these cell–cell protein linkages, the zonula adherens, and the combination of the two junctional arrays means that a relatively impermeable cell layer is formed with minimal paracellular permeability. Changes to these junctional complexes can be expected to occur rapidly whenever superficial cells die or degenerate and are then lost from the ocular surface (Wolosin and Wang, 1995).

Modern research reveals two inter-related ways in which a cell can normally die, namely necrosis or apoptosis (Allen *et al.*, 1997). The former is the commonly accepted one with desquamating cells being described as necrotic, e.g. after being induced to exfoliate by saline irrigation (Begley *et al.*, 1998). This process includes progressive deterioration and eventual lysis of the plasma membrane allowing cytoplasmic contents, including enzymes, to leak out. The necrotic cells will be shed into the tear film and some of them end up on the marginal zone of the eyelid. However, some of the cells can undergo what is called a programmed cell death, also known as apoptosis. In this process, it is the cell nucleus that changes (leading to the production of degraded DNA) without major alteration to the cytoplasmic organelles or the general deterioration of the cytoplasmic membrane. Indeed, a unique characteristic of apoptotic cells is that the cell plasma membrane forms blebs or buds and small anuclear fragments of cells are produced (Allen *et al.*, 1997). A small number of these can be detected on the ocular surface as cell fragments (Ren and Wilson, 1996). Apoptotic cells may also be found in the deeper lying cells of the corneal epithelium and they have different cytoplasmic features when viewed by TEM (Glaso *et al.*, 1993).

TEM studies have provided a range of images of bulbar conjunctival cells, especially with respect to the cell–cell interfaces, but they are otherwise unremarkable cuboidal cells interspersed with large numbers of mature goblet cells (Srinivastan *et al.*, 1977; Kessler *et al.*, 1995; Nichols, 1996). The bulbar conjunctiva is formed into distinct creases, the palisades of Vogt (Lawrenson and Ruskell, 1991), with part of the architecture of the palisades being due to a series of discrete arrays of conjunctival cells that form 'pegs' into the underlying substantia propria. In other parts, some of these creases and folds may even form distinct 'crypts' that are lined with goblet cells because the surface is an invagination of the bulbar surface.

Two special populations of cells, the stem cells, are found in the basal layers. These are considered to play a pivotal role in determining the rate at which the epithelial cells differentiate and mature. Using special antibody-labelling techniques, populations of stem cells have been detected at both the limbal epithelial arcade and at the fornix (Wei *et al.*, 1995; Wolosin and Wang, 1995). The stem cells undergo a unique cell division process in that they essentially divide to produce the equivalent of another stem cell and a daughter cell. The daughter cells divide over and over again and migrate to the basal edge of the corneal epithelium where they can undergo repeated horizontal and vertical mitosis to generate new basal cells and/or intermediate cells (Wolosin and Wang, 1995). A similar process would presumably occur at the fornix.

The meibomian glands are under the tarsal conjunctiva and, in man, are embedded within the collagenous connective tissue of the tarsal plate (Bron et al., 1985). TEM reveals the holocrine structure of the glandular tissue. In man, the meibomian glands are some 4.8 mm long, oriented perpendicular to the eyelid margin and comprise an estimated 32 individual upper glands and 25 individual lower glands (Greiner et al., 1998). A rich and multi-neurotransmitter innervation in the close proximity to these tarsal glands presumably plays a role in controlling secretion during periods of eyelid inactivity or hyperactivity.

The goblet cells are found across the entire surface of the bulbar, fornix, orbital and tarsal conjunctiva (Takakusaki, 1969; Huang et al., 1988; Nichols, 1996; Doughty, 1997). The cells have a 'goblet' shape and are actually individual cells with their own nucleus. The cells start developing in the basal layers and migrate to the surface either singly, in discrete groups or large numbers, with some marked species differences being apparent (Gipson and Tisdale, 1997). Each goblet cell is holocrine and contains hundreds of small 'granules' (packets) of mucus which are expelled out onto the ocular surface through small (7–16 µm wide) oval-shaped orifices (Doughty, 1997). The mucus is not homogeneous and can be of the neutral or acidic type (Huang et al., 1988). Multi-neuro-transmitter innervation is evident in the vicinity of the goblet cells, suggestive of a regulatory role in secretion (Dartt et al., 1995). It has yet to be established whether the stimulus to secrete is stimulatory or nociceptive, whether different types of mucus could be released overall and how any type of secreted mucus is integrated into the ocular surface.

The goblet cells are by no means the only source of ocular surface mucus (Gipson and Inatomi, 1997). Thousands of superficial cells across the palpebral conjunctiva (Greiner et al., 1980; Dilly, 1985; Bergmanson et al., 1999) contain minute vesicles or electron dense granules. The vesicles are thought to be empty granules, with the secretion being mucoid in nature (Rohen and Steuhl, 1982; Dilly, 1985; Gipson and Inatomi, 1997). These 'type II' cells have been known for many years and their large numbers indicate they could contribute significant quantities of different types of mucus to the ocular surface compared to the goblet cells (Gipson and Inatomi, 1997).

A third source of glycoprotein material, presumably in addition to serous (watery) secretions, is the tarsal accessory lacrimal glands. Both the accessory fornix glands of Krause and the accessory tarsal glands of

Wolfring (Gillette *et al.*, 1980; Seifert and Spitznas, 1994; Hunt *et al.*, 1996; Bergmanson *et al.*, 1999) are made up of an acinar arrangement, which is similar to that of the main orbital lacrimal glands (Dartt, 1994). As in the main lacrimal glands, the cells surrounding the acini are connected by series of tight junctions (Hunt *et al.*, 1996; Bergmanson *et al.*, 1999), indicating watery fluid secretion. Both nerve endings and nerve support (myoepithelial) cells can be found around the accessory glands (Seifert and Spitznas, 1994). An extensive network of ductiles underlying the ocular surface emanates from the tarsal accessory lacrimal glands of Wolfring and the cells lining these ductiles are packed with a range of granules which presumably contain mucus-like material. These granules are distinctly different from those found in the goblet cells, but have some resemblance to those seen in type II cells (Bergmanson *et al.*, 1999). The ducts from the tarsal accessory gland of Wolfring are thought to open onto the tarsal/orbital surface at large orifices that can be over 100 μm in diameter (Doughty, 1997; Bergmanson *et al.*, 1999). An extensive net-like system of ducts was visualized in flat mounts of the upper eyelid many years ago (Kessing, 1968) and it seems likely that these recent findings are of the same, often-overlooked system. With the size of the ductile openings and the overall density (Doughty, 1997), the relative contribution of these secretions to the tear film could also be considerable.

One last source of ocular secretions is the mast cell. Within the substantia propria below the bulbar and tarsal conjunctiva are mast cells (Takakusaki, 1969; Srinivastan *et al.*, 1977), as well as the conjunctival (perilimbal) vasculature. Mast cells characteristically contain large numbers of electron-lucent or electron-dense secretory granules (Takakusaki, 1969; Irani, 1997). The granules contain histamine and other amines, and the mast cell can also release enzymes such as tryptase, chymase, cathepsins, carboxypeptidases and perhaps certain esterases (Irani, 1997). In the healthy eye, mast cells do not normally seem to be present within the surface epithelia. However, as inflammation develops mast cells can migrate from the underlying connective tissue into the epithelia. In such a position it is more likely that the secretory products will end up in the tear film as a result of mast cell degranulation.

Origins of the tear film components from the ocular surface

Arguments can be forwarded that there are a number of ways in which the various parts of the ocular surface make specific and non-specific contributions to the composition of the preocular tear film. There are essentially six aspects to this contribution (Bron *et al.*, 1985). These must be considered when an inflammatory response of the conjunctival surface develops.

Much attention has, quite correctly, been given to the composition of the lacrimal fluids, especially those from the main lacrimal glands. It has been well established that the serous fluids contain a mixture of ions and proteins (Dartt, 1994). Notwithstanding such often-described composition, it is an inescapable fact that the lacrimal glands alone are not responsible for the composition of the tear film (Table 1.2).

It is unknown whether healthy superficial corneal epithelial cells make any specific contribution to the tear film. However, with a natural (nightly) cycle of cell desquamation, the cellular debris and the cell constituents will be added to the tear film, perhaps contributing to the significant difference in tear film composition after eyelid closure (Baum, 1997), especially if there is the added stress of overnight contact lens wear. Healthy bulbar conjunctival cells do not show an obvious desquamation cycle although these cells can clearly respond to stress and trauma (e.g. dry eyes, irritation, allergy, contact lens wear) and will degenerate, again adding their constituents to the tear film.

The main contribution that the bulbar conjunctiva makes to the tear film is mucus. The bulbar conjunctival epithelium, especially the nasal zone, contains many goblet cells and so their secretions will logically be added to the tear film. Similarly, most zones of the

Table 1.2 Tear film constituents

From lacrimal glands	From ocular surface
Ions (Na^+, K^+, Mg^{2+}, Ca^{2+}, SO_4^{2-}, PO_4^{2-}, HCO_3^-)	Normal cell debris from natural cell exfoliation
Constitutive secretory proteins (IgA)	Extra cell debris from stress, allergic or cytotoxic insult
Secretory proteins from granules (lysozyme, lactoferrin, peroxidase, lipocalin)	Mucus-like macromolecules from cells
Other proteins (IgE, IgM, serum albumin, pre-albumin)	Metabolites, proteins and mediators from the vasculature
Nutritional factors? (peptides, vitamins)	Inflammatory mediators from mast cells
	Inflammatory mediators from white blood cells

palpebral conjunctiva do not appear to be squamous, although clearly the cells can also show a very pronounced inflammatory response. In normal conditions, the palpebral conjunctiva will add mucus and oils to the tear film from the goblet cells, other cellular secretory sites and the meibomian glands. The dual mucous secretion (goblet cells and cell vesicles) can be expected from the epithelia covering orbital and tarsal zones of the palpebral conjunctiva, although it has yet to be determined whether the mucus from the two sources is the same, similar or completely different.

In the normal healthy conjunctiva, the underlying inflammatory cells (mast cells and Langerhans cells) and the vasculature would not be expected to contribute much to the tear film. However, as soon as the ocular surface reacts to a wide range of stimuli, numerous other components will be added to the tear film. Proteins (e.g. pre-albumin) leak out of the dilated vasculature along with metabolites such as glucose and lactate and are detectable in the tear film. A range of inflammatory mediators (histamine, prostaglandins, substance P, interleukins) can be derived from the vasculature, the stressed cells and from the mast cells under the conjunctiva (Bron *et al.*, 1985). Within just an hour or so of inflammation developing, significant contributions from white blood cells can also be expected (Millichamp and Dziezyc, 1991). It is reasonable to expect that some form of hierarchy exists that determines which mediators are released first and which then stimulate the release of other mediators and macromolecules (Doughty and Bergmanson, 1999).

Summary

The ocular surface is heterogeneous and even histological examination reveals differences in cell stratification. Several types of microscopy *ex vivo* or *in vivo* (with or without the added presence of fluorescein) reveal that the ocular surface should not simply be considered as a layer of cells. The cells differ in size, surface characteristics (microplicae versus microvilli) and junctional arrangements, and also show evidence of distinct organization into domains. However, the significance of these collective features with respect to the overlying tear film remain to be established. Some cells are prone to desquamation and these cells end up in the tear film as debris. Non-epithelial cells (e.g. goblet cells) contribute to the tear film, as does the output from epithelial mucous secretory cells and the meibomian glands. Underlying the ocular surface are the mast cells and the vasculature, both of which can also make significant contributions to the composition and stability of the over-lying tear film.

References

Allen, R. T., Hunter, W. J. and Agrawal, D. K. (1997) Morphological and biochemical characterization and analysis of apoptosis. *J. Pharmacol. Toxicol. Methods*, **37**, 215–228.

Baum, J. L. (1997) Prolonged eyelid closure is a risk to the cornea. *Cornea*, **16**, 602–611.

Begley, C. G., Zhou, J. and Wilson, G. (1998) Characterization of cells shed from the ocular surface of normal eyes. In *Lacrimal Gland, Tear Film, and Dry Eye Syndromes 2* (eds D. A. Sullivan, D. A. Dartt and M. A. Meneray), London, Plenum Press, pp. 675–681.

Bergmanson, J. P. G., Doughty, M. J. and Blocker, Y. (1999) The acinar and ductal organisation of the tarsal accessory lacrimal gland of Wolfring. *Exp. Eye Res.*, **68**, 411–421.

Bitton, E. and Lovasik, J. V. (1998) Longitudinal analysis of precorneal tear film rupture patterns. In *Lacrimal Gland, Tear Film, and Dry Eye Syndromes 2* (eds D. A. Sullivan, D. A. Dartt and M. A. Meneray), London, Plenum Press, pp. 381–389.

Blades, K. and Doughty, M. J. (2000) Comparison of grading schemes to quantitative assessments of nucleus-to-cytoplasmic rations for human bulbar conjunctival cells collected by impression cytology. *Curr. Eye Res.*, **20**, 335–340.

Blades, K., Doughty, M. J. and Patel, S. (1998) Pilot study on the use of impression cytology specimens for quantitative assessment of the surface area of bulbar conjunctival cells. *Optom. Vis. Sci.*, **75**, 591–599.

Bron, A. J., Mengher, L. S. and Davey, C. C. (1985) The normal conjunctiva and its response to inflammation. *Trans. Ophthalmol. Soc. UK*, **104**, 424–435.

Bruckner, R., Batschelet, E. and Hugenschmidt, F. (1987) The Basel longitudinal study on aging (1955–1978). Ophthalmo-gerontological research results. *Doc. Ophthalmol.*, **64**, 235–310.

Dartt, D. A. (1994) Regulation of inositol phosphates, calcium and protein kinase C in the lacrimal gland. *Prog. Retinal Eye Res.*, **13**, 443–478.

Dartt, D. A., McCarthy, D. M., Mercer, H. J. *et al.* (1995) Localization of nerves adjacent to goblet cells in rat conjunctiva. *Curr. Eye Res.*, **14**, 993–1000.

Dilly, P. N. (1985) Contribution of the epithelium to the stability of the tear film. *Trans. Ophthalmol. Soc. UK*, **104**, 381–389.

Doughty, M. J. (1990) A morphometric analysis of the surface cells of rabbit corneal epithelium by scanning electron microscopy. *Am. J. Anat.*, **189**, 316–328.

Doughty, M. J. (1992) Twice-daily use of a chlorobutanol-preserved artificial tear on rabbit corneal epithelium assessed by scanning electron microscopy. *Ophthal. Physiol. Optics*, **12**, 457–466.

Doughty, M. J. (1995) Evaluation of the effects of saline versus bicarbonate containing mixed salts solutions on rabbit corneal epithelium in vitro. *Ophthal. Physiol. Optics*, **15**, 585–599.

Doughty, M. J. (1996a) Evidence for heterogeneity in a small squamous cell type (light cells) in the rabbit corneal epithelium – a scanning electron microscope study. *Doc. Ophthalmol.*, **92**, 117–136.

Doughty, M. J. (1996b) Diagnostic and therapeutic pharmaceutical agents for use in contact lens practice. In *Clinical Contact Lens Practice* (eds E. Bennett and B. A. Weissman), Philadelphia, Lippincott-Raven, pp. 1–38.

Doughty, M. J. (1997) Scanning electron microscopy of the tarsal and orbital conjunctival surfaces compared to peripheral corneal epithelium in pigmented rabbits. *Doc. Ophthalmol.*, **93**, 345–371.

Doughty, M. J. and Fong, W. K. (1992) Topographical differences in cell area at the surface of the corneal epithelium of the pigmented rabbit. *Curr. Eye Res.*, **11**, 1129–1136.

Doughty, M. J. and Panju, Z. (1995) Exploring the hidden surface of the underside of the eyelid. *Cont. Lens Spect.*, **10(7)**, 19–30.

Doughty, M. J. and Bergmanson, J. P. G. (1999) Reassessment of the conjunctival ocular surface of the muco-cutaneous boundary and the ultrastructural search for Marx's line. *Optom. Vis. Sci.*, **76**, 167–178.

Doughty, M. J., Potvin, R., Pritchard, N. and Fonn, D. (1995) Evaluation of the range of areas of the fluorescein staining patterns of the tarsal conjunctiva in man. *Doc. Ophthalmol.*, **89**, 355–371.

Doughty, M. J., Blades, K., Button, N. F. and Wilson, G. S. (2000) Further analysis of the size and shape of cell obtained by impression cytology from the exposed portion of the human bulbar conjunctiva. *Ophthal. Physiol. Opt.*, **20**, 391–400.

Ehlers, N. (1970) Morphology and histochemistry of the corneal epithelium of mammals. *Acta Anat.*, **75**, 161–198.

Fonn, D., Pritchard, N., Garnett, B. and Davids, L. (1996) Palpebral aperture sizes of rigid and soft contact lens wearers compared to non-wearers. *Optom. Vis. Sci.*, **73**, 211–214.

Fox, S. A. (1966) The palpebral fissure. *Am. J. Ophthalmol.*, **62**, 73–78.

Gillette, T. F., Allansmith, M. R., Geiner, J. V. and Janusz, M. (1980) Histologic and immunohistologic comparison of main and accessory lacrimal tissue. *Am. J. Ophthalmol.*, **89**, 724–730.

Gipson, I. K. and Inatomi, T. (1997) Mucin genes expressed by the ocular surface epithelium. *Prog. Retinal Eye Res.*, **16**, 81–98.

Gipson, I. K. and Tisdale, A. S. (1997) Visualization of conjunctival goblet cell actin cytoskeleton and mucin content in tissue whole mounts. *Exp. Eye Res.*, **65**, 407–415.

Glaso, M., Sandvig, K. U. and Haaskjold, E. (1993) Apoptosis in the rat corneal epithelium during regeneration. *APMIS*, **101**, 914–922.

Goller, Th. and Weyrauch, K. D. (1993) Das Konjunktivepithel des Hundes. Licht-und elektronenmikroskopische Untersuchungen. *Annals Anat.*, **75**, 127–134.

Greiner, J. V., Kenyon, K. R., Henriquez, A. S. and Korb, D. R. (1980) Mucus secretory vesicles in conjunctival epithelial cells of wearers of contact lenses. *Arch. Ophthalmol.*, **98**, 1843–1846.

Greiner, J. V., Leahy, C. D., Welter, D. A. *et al.* (1997) Histopathology of the ocular surface after eye rubbing. *Cornea*, **16**, 327–332.

Greiner, J. V., Glonek, T., Korb, D. R. *et al.* (1998). Volume of the human and rabbit meibomian gland system. In *Lacrimal Gland, Tear Film, and Dry Eye Syndromes 2* (eds D. A. Sullivan, D. A. Dartt and M. A. Meneray), London, Plenum Press, pp. 339–343.

Huang, A. J. W., Tseng, S. C. G. and Kenyon, K. R. (1988) Morphogenesis of rat conjunctival goblet cells. *Invest. Ophthalmol. Vis. Sci.*, **29**, 969–975.

Hunt, S., Spitznas, M., Seifert, P. and Rauwolf, M. (1996) Organ culture of human main and accessory lacrimal glands and their secretory behaviour. *Exp. Eye Res.*, **62**, 541–554.

Hymes, C. (1929) The postnatal growth of the cornea and palpebral tissue and the projection of the eyeball in early life. *J. Comp. Neurol.*, **48**, 415–440.

Irani, A.-M. A. (1997) Ocular mast cells and mediators. *Immunol. Allergy Clin. N. Am.*, **17**, 1–18.

Kessing, S. V. (1968) The mucus gland system of the conjunctiva. *Acta Ophthalmol.*, **95(Suppl.)**, 1–19.

Kessler, T. L., Mercer, H. J., Zieske, J. D. *et al.* (1995) Stimulation of goblet cell mucous secretion by activation of nerves in the rat conjunctiva. *Curr. Eye Res.*, **14**, 985–992.

Knop, E. and Brewitt, H. (1992) Induction of conjunctival epithelial alterations by contact lens wearing. A prospective study. *German J. Ophthalmol.*, **1**, 125–134.

Lange, W., Debbage, P. L., Basting, C. and Gabius, H. J. (1989) Neoglycoprotein binding distinguishes distinct zones in the epithelia of the porcine eye. *J. Anat.*, **166**, 243–252.

Laurent, J. and Wilson, G. (1997) Size of cells collected from normal human subjects using contact lens cytology. *Optom. Vis. Sci.*, **74**, 280–287.

Lawrenson, J. G. and Ruskell, G. (1991) The structure of corpuscular nerve endings in the limbal conjunctiva of the human eye. *J. Anat.*, **177**, 75–84.

Millichamp, N. J. and Dziezyc, J. (1991) Mediators of ocular inflammation. *Prog. Vet. Comp. Ophthalmol.*, **1**, 41–58.

Nichols, B. A. (1996) Conjunctiva. *Microsc. Res. Techn.*, **33**, 296–319.

Potvin, R. J., Doughty, M. J. and Fonn, D. (1994) Tarsal conjunctival morphometry of asymptomatic soft contact lens wearers and non-lens wearers. *Int. Contact Lens Clinic*, **21**, 225–231.

Ren, H. and Wilson, G. (1996) Apoptosis in the corneal epithelium. *Invest. Ophthalmol. Vis. Sci.*, **37**, 1017–1025.

Rivas, L., Oroza, M. A., Perez-Esteban, A. and Murube-de-Castillo, J. (1992) Morphological changes in ocular surface in dry eyes and other disorders by impression cytology. *Graef. Arch. Clin. Exp. Ophthalmol.*, **230**, 329–334.

Rohen, J. W. and Steuhl, P. (1982) Specialized cell types and their regional distribution in the conjunctival epithelium of the Cynomolgus monkey. *Graef. Arch. Clin. Exp. Ophthalmol.*, **218**, 59–63.

Rolando, M. and Refojo, M. F. (1983) Tear evaporimeter for measuring water evaporation rate from the tear film under controlled conditions in humans. *Exp. Eye Res.*, **36**, 25–33.

Seifert, P. and Spitznas, M. (1994) Demonstration of nerve fibres in human accessory lacrimal glands. *Graef. Arch. Clin. Exp. Ophthalmol.*, **232**, 107–114.

Smith, P. (1890) On the size of the cornea in relation to age, sex, refraction, and primary glaucoma. *Trans. Ophthalmol. Soc. UK*, **10**, 68–78.

Sotoyama, M., Villanueva, M. B. G., Jonai, H. and Saito, S. (1995) Ocular surface area as an informative index of visual ergonomics. *Indust. Health*, **33**, 43–56.

Srinivastan, B. D., Worgul, B. V., Iwamoto, T. and Merriam, G. R. (1977) The conjunctival epithelium. II. Histochemical and ultrastructural studies on the human and rat conjunctiva. *Ophthalmic Res.*, **9,** 65–79.

Sugrue, S. P. and Zieske, J. D. (1997) ZO1 in corneal epithelium: association to the zonulata occludens and adherens junctions. *Exp. Eye Res.*, **64,** 11–20.

Takakusaki, I. (1969) Fine structure of the human palpebral conjunctiva with special reference to the pathological changes in vernal conjunctivitis. *Arch. Histol. Japan*, **30,** 247–282.

Tiffany, J. M., Todd, B. S. and Baker, M. R. (1998) Computer-assisted calculation of exposed area of the human eye. In *Lacrimal Gland, Tear Film, and Dry Eye Syndromes 2* (eds D. A. Sullivan, D. A. Dartt and M. A. Meneray), London, Plenum Press, pp. 433–439.

Tseng, S. C. G. and Zhang, S.-H. (1995) Interaction between rose bengal and different protein components. *Cornea*, **14,** 427–435.

Watsky, M. A., Jablonski, M. M. and Edelhauser, H. F. (1988) Comparison of conjunctival and corneal surface areas in rabbit and human. *Curr. Eye Res.*, **7,** 483–486.

Wei, Z.-G., Cotsarelis, G., Sun, T.-T. and Lavker, R. M. (1995) Label-retaining cells are preferentially located in fornical epithelium: Implications on conjunctival epithelial homeostasis. *Invest. Ophthalmol. Vis. Sci.*, **36,** 236–246.

Weyruach, K. D. (1983) The conjunctival epithelium in domestic ruminants. I. Light microscopic investigations. *Z. Mikrosk.-anat. Forsch.*, **97,** 585–572.

Williams, K. K. and Watsky, M. A. (1996) Dye spread through gap junctions in the corneal epithelium of the rabbit. *Curr. Eye Res.*, **16,** 445–452.

Wilson, G., Ren, H. and Laurent, J. (1995) Corneal epithelial surface staining. *J. Am. Optom. Assoc.*, **66,** 435–441.

Wolff, E. (1964) The mucocutaneous junction of lid margin and the distribution of tear fluid. *Trans. Ophthalmol. Soc. UK*, **66,** 291–308.

Wolosin, J. M. and Wang, Y. (1995) α-2,3 sialylation differentiate the limbal and corneal epithelial cell phenotypes. *Invest. Ophthalmol. Vis. Sci.*, **36,** 2277–2286.

Zaman, M. L., Doughty, M. J. and Button, N. F. (1998) The exposed ocular surface and its relationship to spontaneous eyeblink rate in elderly Caucasians. *Exp. Eye Res.*, **67,** 681–686.

2 Structure and function of the preocular tear film

Jennifer Craig

Introduction

The tear film is a highly specialized and carefully structured moist film which covers the bulbar and palpebral conjunctivae and the cornea. Quantitatively and qualitatively, its composition must be maintained within fairly narrow limits to maintain a healthy and functional visual system. Abnormalities of the film, affecting the constituents or the volume, can rapidly result in serious dysfunction of the eyelids and conjunctiva and ultimately affect the transparency of the cornea (Records, 1979).

The presence of a healthy tear film is important for four main reasons (Milder, 1987). Firstly, it fills in small surface irregularities in the corneal epithelium, thereby providing a perfect, smooth, regular optical surface. Secondly, the tear film is important mechanically, adhering to the palpebral and bulbar conjunctival surfaces and keeping them moist and well-lubricated. Tears constantly flow across the ocular surface because of the blinking mechanism, and this flushes cellular debris and foreign matter towards the caruncle for elimination. In addition, where an osmotic gradient exists, water can move between the cornea and tear film due to the osmotic pressure. Thirdly, since the corneal surface is avascular, it is highly dependent on the tear film for its nutrition. Oxygen from the ambient air dissolves in the tear fluid and is transferred to the corneal epithelium. Furthermore, nutrients such as glucose, which are found in the bloodstream, are passed from the palpebral conjunctival vessels into the tear film and, again, are transferred to the cornea. Finally, the tear film is the first line of defence against ocular surface infection. This is achieved primarily by the antibacterial activity of certain constituent proteins and enzymes, the principal one being lysozyme.

The tear film forms the marginal tear strips and covers the palpebral conjunctiva, the bulbar conjunctiva and the cornea. For the purposes of clinical examination, the most relevant portion of the tear film is that covering the exposed ocular surface; in particular, the precorneal tear film.

Of the total volume of tear fluid within the palpebral aperture, around 70–90 per cent is found within the marginal tear strips (Mishima *et al.*, 1966; Kwok, 1984; Port and Asaria, 1990). A small proportion lies beneath the eyelids between the palpebral and bulbar conjunctivae, and the remainder covers the cornea and the exposed bulbar conjunctiva. The average thickness of the tear film over the exposed ocular surface varies from approximately 9 µm immediately after a blink, to around 4 µm just before the next blink (Mishima, 1965; Norn, 1969a; Holly, 1981a). The tear film is thinnest immediately adjacent to the marginal tear strip as shown in Figure 2.1. Tear fluid drains from the eye through the puncta which are apposed to the globe, one on each lid margin, near the inner canthus (Wolff, 1946).

A contact lens placed before the cornea, to correct refractive error, is bathed in the preocular tear fluid. For successful contact lens wear, the relationship between the contact lens material, the tear film and the cornea must be harmonious. Dry eye problems are responsible for a high proportion of contact lens failures; therefore, it is important to understand the effect of contact lenses on the tear film, in order that the most suitable lens material and parameters can be chosen.

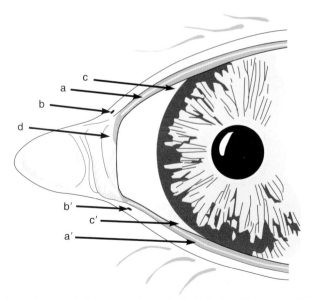

Figure 2.1 The visual axis is directed medially, bringing the corneal limbus within about 3 mm of the caruncle. The upper and lower lids are retracted slightly to show the puncta. a and a' indicate the marginal tear strips; b and b' denote the everted upper and lower puncta; c and c' denote the bands of thinnest tear film; and d denotes the medial lacrimal lake

The healthy tear film is a relatively versatile structure which, to some extent, can adapt to the changing environment. However, in the presence of a disruptive element such as a contact lens, the tear film is unable to maintain its carefully ordered structure and exhibits a fragility which can compromise its health and function. Contact lenses alter the structure, composition, physicochemical properties and dynamic behaviour of the normal tear film (Tomlinson, 1992). Reference will therefore be made throughout this chapter, while describing the structure and function of the normal tear film, to the effect of contact lenses on the various layers and biophysical parameters.

Structure of the tear film

The normal tear film is classically described as a trilaminar structure comprising a superficial lipid layer, an intermediate aqueous phase and an underlying mucous layer (Wolff, 1946; Holly and Lemp, 1977) as illustrated in Figure 2.2.

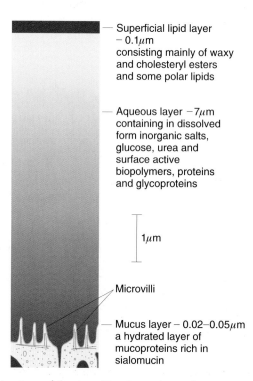

Superficial lipid layer
-0.1μm
consisting mainly of waxy
and cholesteryl esters
and some polar lipids

Aqueous layer -7μm
containing in dissolved
form inorganic salts,
glucose, urea and
surface active
biopolymers, proteins
and glycoproteins

1μm

Microvilli

Mucus layer $-0.02-0.05\mu$m
a hydrated layer of
mucoproteins rich in
sialomucin

Figure 2.2 The structure of the tear film drawn to scale

More recently, investigators have shown that the tear film is more complex than originally believed, containing additional layers and interfaces. Tiffany (1988) proposed a new tear film model which included several interposing, interfacial layers, as shown in Figure 2.3. Prydal *et al.* (1992, 1993) later suggested that previous reports had vastly underestimated the thickness of mucus and proposed that the tear film was around 40 μm instead of 7 μm, with additional mucus providing the difference in thickness. This value has since been disputed (O'Leary and Wilson, 1993), but problems inherent in viewing this layer (due to the similarity in refractive index between the aqueous and mucin layers) make thickness measurements very difficult. Recent work has demonstrated a thickness of between 1.6 and 7.3 μm as determined by reflectance spectra, but is unable to confirm, at this stage, whether this corresponds to the aqueous component alone, or to the entire tear film (King-Smith *et al.*, 1998, 1999). The search for an indisputable value for the thickness of the precorneal tear film therefore continues. Research has also shown that there are dissolved mucins throughout the aqueous phase, decreasing in concentration towards the lipid layer (Dilly, 1994). In fact, it has been suggested that the mucous and aqueous layers should not be considered as completely distinct layers but rather as phases of the tear film, with more or less mucus respectively.

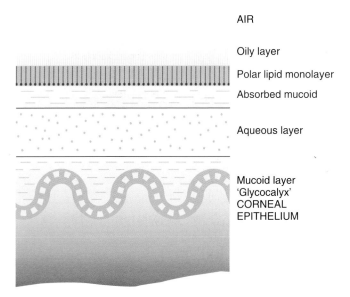

AIR

Oily layer

Polar lipid monolayer

Absorbed mucoid

Aqueous layer

Mucoid layer
'Glycocalyx'
CORNEAL
EPITHELIUM

Figure 2.3 A six-layer model of the tear film showing additional layers and interfaces

Layers of the tear film

The lipid layer

Origin and innervation

The superficial lipid layer is a relatively thin, oily layer, around 100 nm in thickness, and is derived from three sources, all of which are in the eyelids (Figure 2.4). The majority of lipid is produced by the tubulo-acinar meibomian glands, embedded in the upper and lower tarsal plates (Bron and Tiffany, 1998). The blinking action fills and releases meibomian gland fluid from the ducts. Meibomian gland secretion is achieved through a holocrine mechanism, with the entire cell and its lipid content being released (Sirigu *et al.*, 1992). Innervation of the meibomian glands is not fully understood but recent work has indicated that the glands, and the vessels associated closely with them, are richly innervated by both sympathetic and parasympathetic nerve fibres (Chung *et al.*, 1996; Perra *et al.*, 1996). Hormonal control is believed to play a significant role in the regulation of meibomian fluid secretion.

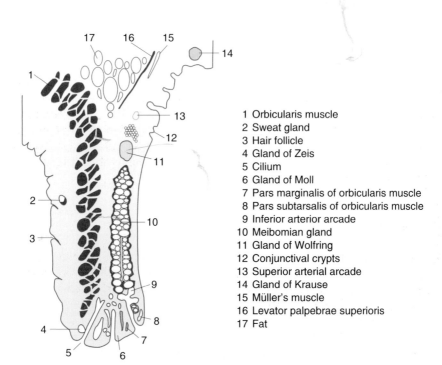

1 Orbicularis muscle
2 Sweat gland
3 Hair follicle
4 Gland of Zeis
5 Cilium
6 Gland of Moll
7 Pars marginalis of orbicularis muscle
8 Pars subtarsalis of orbicularis muscle
9 Inferior arterior arcade
10 Meibomian gland
11 Gland of Wolfring
12 Conjunctival crypts
13 Superior arterial arcade
14 Gland of Krause
15 Müller's muscle
16 Levator palpebrae superioris
17 Fat

Figure 2.4 Sagittal section of the eyelid showing the various glands

The presence of androgen-metabolizing enzymes in the meibomian gland (Perra *et al.*, 1990), and the association between seborrhoeic eczema, a condition known to be influenced by androgen levels (Thody and Shuster, 1979), and meibomian gland dysfunction, has led researchers to believe that a loss in circulating androgens may be a precipitating factor in the development of the disease. Some additional lipid is secreted onto the lid margin by the glands of Moll, and by the lash follicle glands of Zeis (Figure 2.4).

Functions

The lipid layer is important in retarding evaporation of the underlying aqueous layer (Mishima and Maurice, 1961; Iwata *et al.*, 1969; Craig and Tomlinson, 1997). A four-fold increase in tear evaporation is observed when the human lipid layer is absent or is non-confluent (Craig and Tomlinson, 1997). It also prevents contamination of the tear film by skin lipids. This is important since skin lipids differ in composition from tear film lipids and have the potential to destabilize the lipid film (McDonald, 1968). Finally, the lipid forms a barrier which prevents tears from overspilling onto the eyelid (Norn, 1966).

Composition

The lipid layer comprises polar and non-polar lipids. The primary constituents are mixed wax esters and sterol esters. These make up around 90 per cent of the total lipid. The remainder consists of free sterols, free fatty acids, hydrocarbons and phospholipids (Tiffany, 1987). Chromatographic techniques, used to separate and identify the components of the lipid layer, have shown that there is considerable inter-subject variation in tear film lipids (Tiffany, 1978).

Properties

Meibomian oils are seen to spread well over the aqueous phase of the tears in *in vivo* studies (Norn, 1979; Guillon, 1986), but isolated meibomian lipids do not spread well on saline. Meibomian oil melts over a range of temperatures (19–32°C; Tiffany and Marsden, 1986), which are generally within the normal range of eyelid temperatures, although meibomian oil is less fluid than sebum at physiological temperature (Butcher and Coonin, 1949). Human tear lipids are unable to inhibit the evaporation of an underlying saline solution in *in vitro* studies (Brown and Dervichian, 1969). Differences in the findings between *in vivo* and *in vitro* studies are attributed to strong interactions believed to exist between the aqueous tear film components and the lipid layer in the eye, but not when saline is used to mimic the aqueous layer. These interactions are complex and are not fully understood, although a significant role for the tear protein, lipocalin, has been implicated (Schoenwald *et al.*, 1998).

Variations in meibomian oil composition alter the melting point of the lipid layer. This consequently affects the spreading properties and the barrier properties of the layer. An increase in the proportion of high melting point lipids is observed in meibomian keratoconjunctivitis (McCulley and Sciallis, 1977), and is believed to contribute to the poor tear film stability observed in this condition.

Alterations in contact lens wear

The principal alteration to the structure of the tear film, on insertion of a contact lens, is to the superficial lipid layer. In the normal eye, the oily layer is spread over the aqueous phase of the tears by the blink mechanism. Inserting a contact lens on the ocular surface, within the aqueous layer, creates a considerably thinner layer of fluid on which the lipid can lie, and also disturbs the smooth surface over which the lids must sweep during a blink to re-establish the tear film (Guillon, 1986). The combination of these factors results in, at best, a thin lipid layer over a hydrogel contact lens, but the absence of a lipid layer over a rigid contact lens. This difference between the layer over a hydrogel and a rigid lens is related primarily to the relative amounts of movement of the two lens types over the ocular surface during wear.

Similarly, the stability of the tear film is affected in contact lens wear (Guillon and Guillon, 1993; Guillon, 1998). For a stable film to be formed on the surface, the contact lens would be required to be entirely biocompatible with the tear fluid and surrounding tissues, allowing a continuous film, complete with lipid layer, to be formed over the surface. Unfortunately, the relatively hydrophobic nature of contact lens materials, particularly rigid lens materials, often precludes the formation of such a film. Consequently, tear film stability is reduced in the presence of a contact lens. Thick lipid layers are associated with increased tear film stability (Craig *et al.*, 1995). A preocular tear film lipid layer which is thick and stable prior to lens fitting is more likely to form a continuous lipid layer over the surface of a contact lens than one which is thinner and unstable at the outset (Guillon and Guillon, 1993). A lens which can support a continuous lipid layer is more often associated with successful contact lens wear; therefore, it is important to assess tear film structure and stability prior to fitting contact lenses and to monitor these features following fitting. While hydrogel lenses are inherently more wettable than rigid gas permeable lenses, it should be noted that the water content of a hydrogel lens is not directly related to its wettability, since the polymer matrix also plays an important role (Holly, 1979). However, when the contact lens, regardless of the material, is placed on the eye, it quickly becomes covered with a layer of mucus which dramatically improves its wettability (Benjamin *et al.*, 1984). Frequent replacement of contact lenses helps to promote this feature, as deposits on the lens surface are detrimental to the wettability of the lens and cause a reduction in tear film stability (Lowther, 1997).

The aqueous layer

Origin and innervation

The major, intermediate 'watery' phase of the tear film is approximately 6.5–7.5 μm thick (Mishima, 1965) and contains dissolved ions and proteins. The aqueous phase originates from the main lacrimal gland, the accessory glands of Krause and the accessory glands of Wolfring (Milder, 1987).

The lacrimal gland is situated in the superior temporal angle of the orbit and consists of two portions known as the orbital and palpebral lobes. The larger, orbital lobe empties through two to eight ducts into the conjunctival sac mainly at the upper temporal fornix. The ducts of the orbital portion of the gland pass through the smaller palpebral lobe which has 6–10 ducts, such that removal of the palpebral lobe would abolish secretion from the entire lacrimal gland (Milder, 1987).

The human lacrimal gland is a compound tubuloalveolar gland, similar to the salivary gland (Rohen and Lütjen-Drecoll, 1992). Contractile branched myoepithelial cells, which lie between the basal lamina and the acinus cells, surround the endpieces of the lacrimal gland (Figure 2.5). Their precise function in the lacrimal gland has not been established, but such cells can accelerate glandular secretion by spontaneous contraction in other parts of the body (Dartt, 1992). The interstitial tissue of the lacrimal gland is wide-meshed and rich in free cells. These cells are typically eosinophils, lymphocytes, macrophages and plasma cells. The plasma cells contribute to the antibodies in the tear film (IgA), while the remainder arise from the serum through leakage from the conjunctival vessels. A dense network of capillaries around the ducts is thought to aid fluid adsorption.

The concentration of water and solutes produced by the endpieces, is modified as the fluid passes along the lacrimal ducts. Here, water is secreted or absorbed (depending on whether the demand is for basal or reflex tear flow) and potassium ions are secreted into the fluid. Proteins

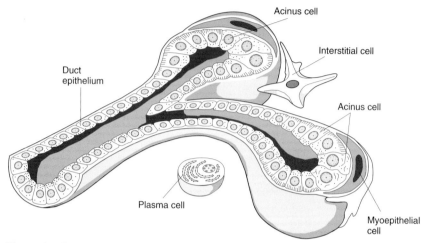

Figure 2.5 Schematic diagram illustrating different cell types in the lacrimal gland

and other substances can also be secreted by the duct cells, but the final tear film composition is not achieved until the fluid from the lacrimal gland is combined with the secretions of the accessory glands, the ocular surface epithelia and the meibomian glands (Dartt, 1992).

Innervational control of tear secretion is derived from the trigeminal nerve (V) (principal afferent pathway), the facial nerve (VII) (principal efferent pathway) and cervical sympathetic nerve fibres (Figure 2.6; Milder, 1987).

The lacrimal gland is responsible for reflex tear secretion. Reflex secretion may be of peripheral sensory origin through trigeminal nerve stimulation (cornea, conjunctiva, skin, nose) or of central sensory origin. In the latter, the stimulation may be retinal, varying with intensity of light, or psychogenic, as in weeping caused by emotional disturbances or by various central nervous system diseases (Milder, 1987).

Neuronal control of lacrimal gland fluid secretion has become more fully understood in recent years. Parasympathetic fibres are intimately disposed around the acinar cells, duct cells, myoepithelial cells and blood vessels. Sympathetic nerves innervate the blood vessels and may be associated with the myoepithelial cells. The parasympathetic nerves primarily control electrolyte/water and protein secretion, by means of the neurotransmitter, acetylcholine, and biologically active peptide, VIP (vasoactive intestinal peptide) (Dartt, 1992). Receptors for the cholinergic agonists are located on the acinar cells, probably on the cells of the duct, and are also found on blood vessels. Stimulation by cholinergic agonists causes vasodilation which increases the rate of secretion. The sympathetic

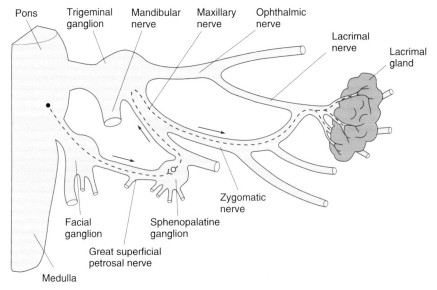

Figure 2.6 Schematic representation of the innervation of the gland

nervous system mainly innervates the lacrimal gland blood vessels, by means of the neurotransmitter, norepinephrine. Other neurotransmitters found in parasympathetic or sympathetic sensory nerve fibres include Substance P, an enkephalin family of peptides, calcitonin gene-related peptide and neuropeptide Y (Dartt, 1992). These are also believed to have potential roles in the control of electrolyte/water and protein secretion.

A proportion of the aqueous component of the tears is also secreted by the accessory lacrimal glands. There are approximately 20 glands of Krause in the upper conjunctival fornix, and around six to eight glands in the lower fornix. Some lacrimal secretion is produced by the glands of Wolfring, which are located mainly in the supratarsal conjunctiva of the upper lid and occasionally in the infratarsal conjunctiva of the lower lid (Figure 2.4; Milder, 1987). Currently, there is no direct evidence to support regulation of the accessory lacrimal glands, but there is indirect evidence in rabbit studies (Gilbard et al., 1990). Such regulation would allow these glands to respond to challenges and alterations in the environment, and help the tear film to remain stable and constant.

Functions

The electrolytes present in the tear film are responsible for the osmolality (tonicity) of the tears (Bothelo, 1964). These essential ions play an important role in maintaining epithelial integrity. Proteins present in the tears also serve many functions. These include a generalized wetting action by lowering the surface tension, and allowing the tear film to spread over and wet the cornea and conjunctival surfaces more effectively. Other important functions include metal transport, control of infectious agents, osmotic regulation, and buffering against changes that would affect equilibrium (Records, 1979).

Composition

The aqueous phase of the healthy preocular tear film contains many ions and molecules including electrolytes, hydrogen ions, proteins, enzymes and metabolites (Milder, 1987).

Electrolytes/hydrogen ions

It has been proposed that basic tear solution contains water, and sodium, potassium, magnesium, calcium, chloride, bicarbonate and phosphate ions. Levels of potassium and chloride ions are greater in tear fluid than in plasma suggesting that they are secreted or concentrated by the lacrimal gland (Milder, 1987). Tear pH is dependent on the concentration of hydrogen ions in the tear fluid.

Proteins/enzymes

More than 60 different components of human tear proteins have been identified (Gachon *et al.*, 1979), but only the major tear proteins (Janssen and van Bijsterveld, 1983) will be described (Table 2.1). The relative proportions of the proteins present in an individual tear sample depend on the method of tear collection (Milder, 1987). Invasive methods, including filter paper and cellulose sponges, stimulate the conjunctiva, induce serum leakage, and result in a higher proportion of plasma proteins. Samples collected by less invasive means, such as fine capillary tubes dipped into the tear meniscus, demonstrate a higher proportion of lacrimal gland proteins. The total protein content of normal basal tears varies from around 0.136–4.5 g/100 ml, with an average of 0.7 g/100 ml (Jaseplson and Lockwood, 1964).

Tear lipocalin is an acidic protein (Fullard and Kissner, 1991) that predominates in tears. The specific function of tear lipocalin has not been

Table 2.1 Major components of human tear proteins	
Lacrimal gland proteins	*Serum proteins*
Lysozyme	Albumin
Lactoferrin	Transferrin
Tear lipocalin	IgG
Secretory IgA	IgM

established, but its amino acid sequence has been identified and found to match closely the lipocalin family of proteins (Redl *et al.*, 1992). It has been shown to be capable of binding and transporting an extensive array of endogenous lipid molecules (Glasgow *et al.*, 1995). It is possible, therefore, that tear lipocalin could bind fatty acid ligands to the outer surface of the tear film and thus contribute significantly to tear film stability. With a deficiency of tear lipocalin it has been considered conceivable that the lipid components could migrate out of the eye by precipitation leading to the formation of mucous strands and disruption of the tear film (Schoenwald *et al.*, 1998). Albumin, identical to serum albumin, forms only a minor component of continuous tears but rises markedly with conjunctival stimulation (Sapse *et al.*, 1969).

Antibodies, which are also known as immunoglobulins, are protein molecules synthesized by plasma cells. They comprise approximately 20 per cent of the total serum protein, but a rather lesser proportion of total (unstimulated) tear protein (Milder, 1987), and are believed to effect the humoral aspects of immunity. In humans there are five distinct immunoglobulin types, each with a specific chemical composition, physical configuration and biological function. They are designated IgA, IgD, IgE, IgG and IgM, on the basis of their immunologic activity and function and they play an important role in ocular defence. Individual immunoglobulins are antigen-specific. Greater amounts of the immuno-globulins, IgE, IgM and IgG, are measured in the tear film in the presence of ocular inflammation (McClellan *et al.*, 1973) or when the conjunctiva is stimulated during tear sample collection since these large immunoglobu-lins originate in the bloodstream. Their presence in the tear film is thus suggestive of serum leakage. IgA, the predominant immunoglobulin of the tears, is attached to an antigenic fragment, secretory component, and has been proposed as the first line of the host defence mechanism by furnishing the conjunctiva with an immunologic coating (Heremans, 1968). Fluorescent antibody and ultrastructural techniques have demonstrated IgA contained within plasma cells in the lacrimal gland, and consequently implicate local production of this immunoglobulin

(Franklin *et al.*, 1973). A plentiful and active immunoglobulin system, combined with active phagocytic cells (e.g. lymphocytes and white blood cells) in the tear film, is important to help protect against invasion of micro-organisms, particularly as the thin, non-keratinized corneal epithelium and abundant blood supply of the conjunctiva increase the susceptibility of the anterior eye to opportunistic infection.

Around 20–40 per cent of the total tear protein is made up of lysozyme (Farris, 1985), the most alkaline protein in the tears. The concentration of lysozyme in the tear film is higher than in any other bodily fluid. It is a long-chain, high-molecular weight, glycolytic enzyme produced by lysosomes (within the cellular ultrastructure). It has the ability to dissolve bacterial walls by enzymatic digestion of tissue muco-polysaccharides (Milder, 1987). Although lysozyme is present in most animal tissues and secretions, its concentration is high enough to be antibacterial only in white blood cells, nasal secretions and tears. Lysozyme levels decrease with age and in dry eye (Seal *et al.*, 1986).

The non-lysozymal bactericidal protein, beta-lysin, is found in tears and aqueous humour (Ford *et al.*, 1976). It is reported to be derived chiefly from platelets, but exists in higher concentration in tears than in blood plasma. Beta-lysin acts primarily on the cellular membrane, in contrast to lysozyme which dissolves bacterial cell walls.

Lactoferrin is an iron-binding protein which occurs in most bodily fluids including saliva, nasal secretions, tears and other biological fluids associated with epithelial surfaces (Farris, 1985). It is produced by the lacrimal gland and therefore its concentration decreases with decreased tear flow accompanying aqueous-deficient dry eye (Seal *et al.*, 1986). Similar to lysozyme, lactoferrin has antibacterial properties. It removes (by binding) the iron necessary for the replication of bacteria. Its action is therefore classed as bacteristatic rather than bactericidal. Transferrin has a similar mode of action to lactoferrin, but is present in much lower concentrations in tears (Aisen and Leibman, 1972). Its presence is a result of passive transport, together with serum proteins, rather than active secretion.

Twelve enzymes have been identified in the tears. These include significant amounts of lactate dehydrogenase (LDH), pyruvate kinase, malate dehydrogenase (MDH), and amylase. These are present in concentrations similar to those in the lacrimal gland, but unlike those in serum (van Haeringen and Glasius, 1974). In conditions of corneal stress, the concentration of LDH increases, while the concentration of MDH does not. The LDH/MDH ratio can thus be used as an index of hypoxic stress (Fullard and Carney, 1985). The ratio has been shown to increase during overnight eye closure, when there is reduced oxygen supply to the ocular surface. The high level of LDH in the tears is found to decrease throughout the first three hours after awakening, to a stable minimum for the remainder of the waking hours (Fullard and Carney, 1984). A similar degree of hypoxic stress to that observed with eye closure is induced during contact lens wear (Fullard and Carney, 1986). Not unexpectedly, the ratio is higher when lenses of lower oxygen permeability, rather than highly oxygen permeable lenses, are fitted.

Metabolites

Tear metabolites include glucose and urea (van Haeringen and Glasius, 1974). The source of these compounds is the blood and they are conveyed to the tear film by a transport system from serum. Higher levels of glucose are observed in the tears following serum-leakage, induced when invasive methods of tear collection are used.

Miscellaneous

There are many other types of cells in the tear film, some living and some dead (Records, 1979). These include fragmented cells from the cornea, the conjunctival epithelium, blood vessels and the conjunctival lymphatic tissues (Norn, 1966). Most of these cells are epithelial cells, lymphocytes or leukocytes. Many become trapped within the mucus beneath the lower lid and are drawn medially towards the caruncle for elimination (Norn, 1969b).

Properties

Normal tear pH values have been quoted as between 7.14 and 7.82 with a mean value, similar to plasma pH, at around 7.4–7.5 (Yamada *et al.*, 1997). It is lowest on wakening as a result of acid byproducts associated with the relatively anaerobic conditions in prolonged eyelid closure, and it increases fairly rapidly due to the loss of CO_2 once the eyes are open (Carney and Hill, 1976). Tear pH is characteristic for each individual, and the normal buffering mechanism (bicarbonate) maintains the pH at a relatively constant level during waking hours (Carney and Hill, 1976). The permeability of the corneal epithelium is thought not to be affected significantly by wide variations in tear pH. However, solutions with a pH below 6.6 or above 7.8 can cause irritation on instillation (Milder, 1987).

Osmolality is an expression of the total concentration of dissolved particles in a solution without regard to their size, density, configuration or electrical charge. Osmolality decreases slightly during overnight eye closure, as a result of decreased tear film evaporation during sleep (Terry and Hill, 1978). Following stabilization of the osmolality on eye-opening, no repeatable diurnal variations have been reported (Craig, 1995a).

Osmolality increases in dry eye (Gilbard et al., 1978) signifying an increased concentration of particles, mainly electrolytes (Bothelo, 1964). Typical increases are shown in Table 2.2 (Craig, 1995b). This can be as a result of increased tear evaporation in the presence of normal tear production (evaporative dry eye) or of aqueous-deficient dry eye.

Table 2.2 Typical increases in tear osmolality in dry eye	
Condition	Expected range of values
Normal	<312 mOsm/kg
Borderline dry eye	312–323 mOsm/kg
Moderate/severe dry eye	>323 mOsm/kg

Some artificial tear supplements (used to alleviate dry eye symptoms) are designed to have a low osmolality, in an attempt to reduce the tear osmolality on application. As intended, the tear osmolality does in fact decrease on instillation, but is found to return to pre-instillation levels within minutes (Holly and Lamberts, 1981; Gilbard and Kenyon, 1985).

Alterations with contact lens wear

An alteration in the rate of tear flow in new contact lens wearers brings about a change in the composition of the tears (Tomlinson, 1992). During adaptation to contact lenses, a reduction in the concentration of electrolytes and serum-derived proteins is observed due to the increase in flow of reflex tears from the lacrimal gland. Another short-term compositional change is in the level of glucose in the tear film during adaptation to hydrogel contact lenses (Kilp, 1978). This is believed to be due to mechanical irritation which causes increased reflex tearing from the lacrimal gland and this, in turn, flushes the glucose from the corneal epithelial cells as a result of the lowered diffusion resistance of the cells. There are few consistent reports in the literature of long-term changes in the tear film composition with contact lens wear, except for IgA levels which have been found to be higher in rigid lens wearers than in hydrogel lens wearers. Again, this is probably due to mechanical stimulation of the conjunctiva and subsequent leakage of serum proteins (Temel *et al.*, 1991).

The influence of contact lens wear on the pH of the tear film is unclear. Some workers claim that there is no alteration in pH whilst others have observed a decrease with contact lens wear (although remaining within normal limits). The minimal changes which occur are testament to the excellent buffering capacity of the tear film (Tomlinson, 1992).

Contact lens wear initially produces a decreased tear osmolality (due to excessive tearing). However, the increased evaporation resulting from disrupted lipid layer during contact lens wear (Tomlinson and Cedarstaff, 1982) is the most probable cause of increased tear osmolality following adaptation. It has been suggested that there may also be decreased tear production corresponding to decreased corneal sensitivity which may contribute to the increased osmolality in adapted contact lens wearers (Gilbard *et al.*, 1986).

The mucous layer

Origin and innervation

The thickness of the deep mucous layer of the tear film remains under debate. The principal sources of mucin are the goblet cells of the conjunctiva (primary source) and the crypts of Henle in the fornices (Figure 2.4). The existence of the glands of Manz in the limbal ring, once believed to be an additional source of mucin (Manz, 1859), was later disproved (Aurell and Kornerup, 1949). It is believed that the structures mistaken for glands in these early studies were, in fact, the limbal palisades. Secondary sources of mucin are the non-goblet epithelial cells of the conjunctiva which contain mucus secretory vesicles (Dilly, 1986). The number of vesicles increases in certain disease states, such as allergic conjunctivitis.

The preocular tear film of the human eye is dependent upon a constant supply of mucus, which must be of adequate chemical and physical quality to maintain the corneal and conjunctival surfaces in the proper state of hydration (Rohen and Lütjen-Drecoll, 1992), as well as to carry out many of the other vital functions of the tears such as lubrication (Kaura and Tiffany, 1986). Mucus is secreted by the goblet cells, of which there are approximately 1.5 million distributed over the conjunctival surface (Figure 2.7; Kessing, 1968). These unicellular glands are most numerous over the nasal conjunctiva and plica and least in the superior temporal bulbar conjunctiva. The mucous layer contains high molecular weight proteins with a high carbohydrate-to-protein ratio, known as glycoproteins.

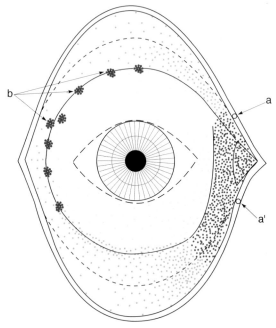

Figure 2.7 The eyelids have been severed from their medial and lateral attachments and are stretched apart schematically exhibiting the entire conjunctival surface of the right eye. The two puncta are indicated by a and a'. The superior and inferior fornices are indicated by the solid concentric lines around the cornea. The crypts of Henle (b) are found in the fornix, mainly superotemporally. The population of mucous glands is indicated by the black dots. They are most concentrated near the plica and inferiorly over the surface of the medial bulbar and inferior palpebral conjunctiva. Their population is least dense in the superior temporal quadrant

Goblet cells are found alone or in groups, located in the surface of the conjunctival epithelium, and connected by tight junctions to neighbouring cells. These specialized apocrine cells (Wanko *et al.*, 1964) produce mucins, which are stored in large secretory granules at the apical side of the cell. The exact mechanism of goblet cell mucin secretion is not fully understood, but is believed to be under neuronal control (Dartt, 1992). Goblet cells are not directly innervated (Kessing, 1968); however, the conjunctival stroma and stratified squamous cells of the epithelium are, allowing a pathway for the diffusion of neurotransmitters to the goblet cells (Ruskell, 1985). It is thought that neurotransmitter ligand-binding to cell surface receptors causes the mucin granule membranes to fuse with the apical goblet cell membrane which releases mucin onto the ocular surface (Dartt, 1994). Such neuronal regulation of secretion could allow for rapid mucin release in response to surface irritants, trauma or to bacterial or environmental toxins (Kessler and Dartt, 1994).

Functions

Ocular mucus performs several functions. Among the most important of these is lubrication, allowing the eyelid margins and palpebral conjunctiva to slide smoothly over one another with minimal friction during blinking and ocular rotational movements (Kaura and Tiffany, 1986). Another important function is protection of the epithelial surfaces. Mucous threads are responsible for covering foreign bodies with a slippery coating of mucus to protect the cornea and conjunctiva from abrasion. Ocular mucus also helps to wet the ocular surface, both directly (Lin and Brenner, 1986) and through the role of the ocular glycoproteins in glycocalyx formation (Dilly, 1994). The corneal surface was originally believed to be hydrophobic in nature (Holly and Lemp, 1971) but more recent studies, using sophisticated techniques, have shown the corneal surface to be relatively wettable and capable of supporting the tear film without the aid of mucus (Tiffany, 1990a, 1990b). However, when areas of non-wetting occur, for example, as a result of epithelial desquamation or surface damage, the mucus may play an essential role in overcoming the temporary hydrophobicity (Tiffany, 1994).

Composition

The goblet cells of the conjunctiva secrete a heterogeneous group of O-linked glycoproteins (Neutra and LeBlond, 1966). These mucins differ in composition from those produced by the subsurface secretory vesicles of the non-goblet conjunctival epithelial cells in normal eyes (Greiner *et al.*, 1979). Dilly proposed that subsurface vesicles are a source of long chain glycoprotein 'binding' molecules (glycocalyx). The vesicles form and migrate to the surface of the cell (Figure 2.8). The vesicle becomes part of the cell membrane and the binding molecules project into the tear film. The subsurface vesicle molecules are thought to bind the mucus from the goblet cells onto the epithelium. The presence of the glycocalyx at the epithelial surface probably renders this area of interface highly polar and, consequently, wettable by aqueous solutions. In diseases of the epithelial cells, this glycocalyx anchoring system is destroyed, with a subsequent destabilization of the tear film (Dilly, 1994).

Properties

The mucus has been shown to be viscoelastic in nature and can respread to heal, rapidly, any gaps or imperfections in its surface (Kaura and Tiffany, 1986). The edges of each surface defect are believed to be brought together by attraction forces, enhanced by the compression of blinking.

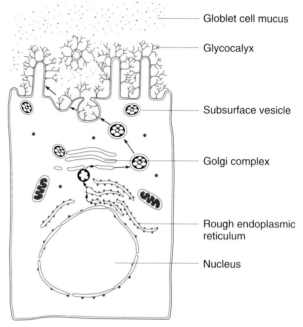

Figure 2.8 Theory of the formation and origin of the glycocalyx of the surface conjunctival cells

The surface of the mucous phase is the first solid layer encountered by invading material such as bacteria, therefore the rapid self-repair of mucous layer imperfections is essential in protecting the epithelium against both localized surface drying effects and bacterial infiltration.

Due to its micellar structure, this layer probably also acts as an immuno-globulin reservoir. It allows slow release of the immunoglobulins over the day, when the open-eye state renders the ocular surface more vulnerable to air-borne pathogens (Dilly, 1994). The intact mucous layer has been demonstrated to reduce *Pseudomonas aeruginosa* adherence to the cornea (Fleiszig *et al.*, 1994). Thus, alterations in mucus production, composition and clearance (as found in some dry eye conditions), and the use of mucolytic agents, may contribute to the pathogenesis of infectious keratitis.

Alterations in contact lens wear

Changes in mucus production have been observed with contact lens wear (Greiner and Allansmith, 1981), conjunctivitis (Takakusaki, 1969) and keratoconjunctivitis sicca (KCS) (Versura *et al.*, 1986). The number of non-goblet epithelial cells increases in both contact lens wear and conjunctivitis, but there is almost a complete absence in advanced KCS (Dilly, 1985). The quantities of several goblet cell mucins have also been found to alter in KCS compared with in normal eyes. In contact lens wearers, no change in the number of goblet cells has been observed, but the composition has been found to alter to include more glycosidic residues, possibly as a response to lens wear (Versura et al., 1986). Such alterations may result in contact lens deposits and, consequently, may be partially responsible for the reduction in tear film stability in contact lens wearers.

Tear production

The basal tear production rate is between 1 and $2\,\mu l/min$ with a turnover rate of approximately 16 per cent per minute in normal subjects (Mishima et al., 1966; Puffer et al., 1980; Wright, 1985). Most researchers have found no diurnal variation in basal tear production (Henderson and Prough, 1950). Anaesthetics have been found to reduce the rate of tear flow; however, despite this, there remains a contribution from the main lacrimal gland as well as from the accessory glands (Jordan and Baum, 1980). Long-term changes in tear production with contact lens wear are not well-documented in the literature, but an initial, short-term increase in the rate of reflex tearing, particularly in rigid gas-permeable contact lens wearers, has been observed, as a result of mechanical irritation during the adaptation phase (Tomlinson, 1992).

Iatrogenic effects on tear production

Several systemic medications have been shown to adversely affect the quantity and/or the quality of the preocular tear film (Doughty, 1997). Hyposecretion of tears is more common than hypersecretion and induces similar symptoms to those experienced with idiopathic dry eye, e.g. grittiness and burning.

Although rarely inducing symptoms, a number of medications have been reported to cause lacrimal gland hyposecretion. The mechanisms by which they do this are not fully understood, however. Medications which can cause such a tear deficiency, and potentially the associated side-effect of dry mouth, include high doses of oral diuretics such as the thiazide diuretics or oral H_1-blocking antihistamines, prescribed primarily for sedation or control of nausea. Drugs with an anti-cholinergic action can have a similar effect on the tear film. Such medications include hysocine-based drugs for gastro-intestinal upset or travel sickness, and tricyclic antidepressants used to combat insomnia. Other drugs indicated for the short-term relief of anxiety or insomnia, the benzodiazepines (including diazepam and nitrazepam), and antipsychotic drugs, such as the phenothiazines, can also cause lacrimal hyposecretion. Additionally, such medications can affect the blink characteristics, altering tear film re-establishment due to the abnormal sweeping action of the eyelids, which can further compromise the preocular tear film.

It should be noted that, since most adverse hyposecretion effects on the lacrimal system are minimal, the *British National Formulary* (*BNF*) or *MIMS* directories of pharmaceuticals may not comment on lacrimal effects *per se*. Thus, when determining adverse reactions to systemic medications, information on anti-cholinergic effects or CNS disturbances should be sought.

Lacrimal secretion may also be reduced with systemic beta-adrenergic blocking drugs (β-blockers) such as propanolol, and it is suspected that this is also true for alpha$_2$-adrenergics, such as the CNS-acting anti-hypertensive medication, oral clonidine. To date, no conclusive evidence exists to show that alpha$_1$-adrenergic drugs alter tear film production.

The above medications are prescribed only if warranted by the general medical condition and, for the most part, management of the medical condition takes precedence over the risk of inducing mild dry eye symptoms. Consequently, it is rare that a medication will be discontinued on the basis of such symptoms, and it may be necessary for the iatrogenic dry eye condition to be managed with artificial tear supplements, during the course of treatment.

True hypersecretion (an increase in tear flow *per se*) is rare, but some medications can cause ocular irritation which results, indirectly, in an increase in tearing due to the reflex tearing. Similarly, the volume of tears in the conjunctival sac may increase, indirectly, as a result of poor tear drainage. Hypersecretion tends to cause symptoms (mild epiphora) which are inconvenient in nature, rather than painful, but can result in reduced tear film stability creating a paradoxical 'wet dry eye'. Some medications for leukaemia (e.g. oral cytarabine or cyclophosphamide) produce a general toxic reaction to the conjunctival membranes and subsequently a chronic irritation which induces reflex tearing.

Treatment for allergy with nasal decongestants can be associated with rebound tear (and nasal) hypersecretion, as the drug wears off between doses or following cessation of the medication. Oral morphine and related compounds are narcotic opioid analgesics and have the potential to cause lacrimal hypersecretion. This same potential exists where anticholinesterases are used, to enhance transmission in neuromuscular disorders such as myasthenia gravis. Significant problems are rare, however, with the majority of affected patients reporting no more than 'moist' eyes.

Some systemic medications do not affect the lacrimal gland and therefore do not alter the aqueous secretion, but they can disrupt the tear film by affecting other components. Isotretinoin is one such drug which affects the meibomian glands and is also believed to affect the conjunctival surface. This could affect both the lipid produced by the meibomian glands in the upper and lower eyelids, and the mucus production from the goblet cells of the conjunctiva. With a deficiency in either of these layers, the tear film would be structurally affected, potentially causing significant tear film instability.

Thus, there are several systemic medications which have the potential to cause alterations to the tear film (Doughty, 1997). In a robust, healthy lacrimal system, few problems may be encountered, but in susceptible individuals, such as those with marginal dry eye or contact lens wearers, the effects of the medication may be sufficient to induce dry eye symptoms. Where the medication cannot be modified, treatment of the iatrogenic dry eye condition may be an appropriate adjunct to the systemic therapy.

Tear film stability

A stable preocular tear film depends on many factors including the correct quantity and quality of the various components of the tears. Measurement of tear stability can provide important information about tear film integrity and function. The mechanism by which the tears destabilize following a blink is not fully understood but several theories have been proposed. Disturbances of the lipid layer result in increased evaporation of the underlying layers but destabilization by this process would take several minutes (Holly, 1981a, 1981b). Since tear break-up generally occurs within a minute of the last blink, evaporation cannot be the sole mechanism. One of the more popular theories, proposed by Holly (1973), suggested that the more rapid break-up of the tears could be attributed to the migration of lipids from the superficial layer towards the mucous layer, contaminating it, and creating small hydrophobic areas which would no longer support the aqueous phase. In the normal eye, the blinking process re-establishes the tear film regularly, preventing break-up occurring. Sharma and Ruckenstein (1985) proposed an alternative mechanism in which van der Waals dispersion forces within the mucous layer were considered to be responsible for the break-up of the tears. Independently, these forces would be insufficient to disrupt the tear film but, together with evaporation and drainage, and disruption of the mucous layer due to interfacial non-homogeneities, the aqueous layer would destabilize in around

15–50 seconds. Other hypotheses have been proposed in which the integrity of the corneal epithelium has been considered to be the major factor in determining tear stability (Liotet *et al.*, 1987). Interference with the ability of the epithelial cells to manufacture glycocalyx (Figure 2.8; Dilly, 1994) is believed to result in insufficient sites for mucous layer attachment.

Tear dynamics and drainage

Elimination of the tears occurs by several routes: through the excretory system (by pumping action and drainage into the nasal passages), by evaporation and by conjunctival absorption.

Excretory system

In the active excretory system, the tears secreted into the upper temporal fornix are conducted towards the lacrimal puncta (Figure 2.9) in three ways (Milder, 1987). At the lateral canthus, the tears move downward, by gravity, to form the lower marginal tear strip. The lower canaliculus is believed to collect four times as much of the tear flow as the upper canaliculus. Capillary attraction helps conduct tears into the punctum and the vertical section of the canaliculus. Finally, lid movement contributes to the movement of tears to the puncta, by the act of blinking. Blinking not only spreads the tear strips over the eye as a film but also moves the tears towards the puncta with each blink. Because the orbicularis muscle is more firmly fixed at its nasal attachment, and the temporal part of the orbicularis ring moves in a nasal direction during blinking, tears are directed nasally with each blink. In addition, the temporal end of the palpebral aperture closes more rapidly as the eyes close in a blink, further contributing to this nasal passage of tears (Milder, 1987). A schematic diagram of the drainage portions of the lacrimal system is shown in Figure 2.9. The direction of the normal flow of tears is indicated by the small arrows.

As the tears enter the lacrimal puncta, they are propelled through the canaliculi into the tear sac by the same blinking movements. Each canaliculus has a short vertical and a longer horizontal segment. Where the two segments join, the canaliculus opens out into an ampulla. Orbicularis fibres are in close contact with the punctum and the canaliculus, so that when this muscle contracts in blinking, the punctum is drawn nasally, the ampulla is compressed, and the horizontal limb of the canaliculus is shortened, forcing tears into the lacrimal sac.

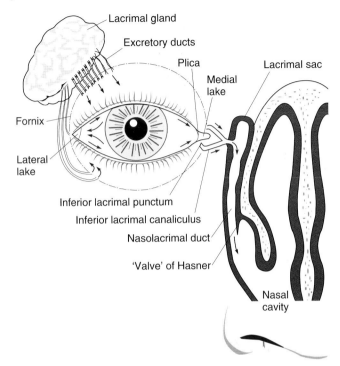

Figure 2.9 A schematic diagram of the secretory and drainage portions of the lacrimal system. The flow of tears is indicated by the small arrows. A general flow in the tear film in the inner palpebral area is towards the lateral lacrimal lake and then along the menisci on the eyelid margins to the puncta

In blinking, the contraction of the orbicularis draws the lateral wall of the sac in a lateral direction. This creates negative pressure and aspirates the tears, forced along the canaliculus by the same orbicularis contraction, into the lacrimal sac. When the orbicularis relaxes after the blink, the sac collapses and this drives the accumulated tears into the nasolacrimal duct (Figure 2.10).

The nasolacrimal duct plays little or no role in the active transport of tears, but the variable folds and valves (including the 'valve' of Hasner) in the duct form a baffle which prevents air currents within the nose from being drawn up into the drainage system (Figure 2.9).

The edge characteristics of a contact lens disrupt the natural blinking process which requires close apposition of the eyelids to the ocular surface. Contact lens wearers have been shown to blink less and to exhibit a higher proportion of incomplete blinks than non-contact lens wearers (Holly, 1981b; Hill, 1984). This serves to reduce the stability of the prelens

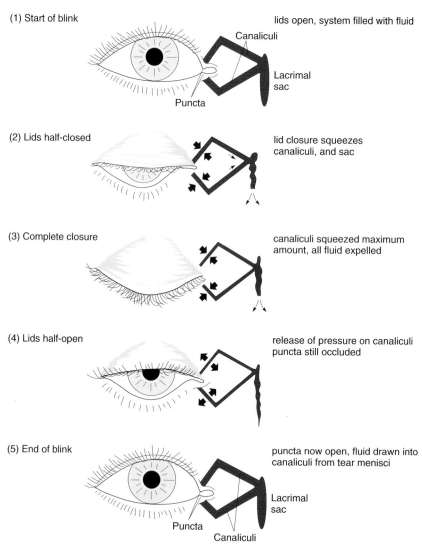

(1) Start of blink — lids open, system filled with fluid
Canaliculi
Lacrimal sac
Puncta

(2) Lids half-closed — lid closure squeezes canaliculi, and sac

(3) Complete closure — canaliculi squeezed maximum amount, all fluid expelled

(4) Lids half-open — release of pressure on canaliculi puncta still occluded

(5) End of blink — puncta now open, fluid drawn into canaliculi from tear menisci
Lacrimal sac
Puncta
Canaliculi

Figure 2.10 The sequence of events in the blink-driven tear drainage process. In (1), the blink has just started and the canaliculi contain tear fluid drawn in immediately following the previous blink. In (2), the lids are half-closed but the puncta are occluded by the abutting lid margins, and the canaliculi and sac are beginning to be compressed. In (3), the lids have reached their point of maximum closure and the canaliculi have been compressed, forcing the contained fluid into and through the sac. In (4), the lids have opened halfway and the pressure on the canaliculi and sac is reduced. The punctal openings are still occluded by the lid margins. In (5), the lids are fully open, the canaliculi and sac expanded to their normal configuration, and tear fluid is drawn into the canaliculi via the punctal openings. This flow typically lasts 1–2 s, by which time the tear fluid in each meniscus is drawn down to its normal level

tear film, highlighting the importance of encouraging such patients to perform blinking exercises.

It should be noted that, in blinking in the normal eye, the lids also play an important role in distributing the fluid evenly over the ocular surface and reforming the tear film. The mechanism involves a biphasic movement. First of all, the eyelid pulls the lipid with it as the eye opens. This oily layer then drags the aqueous layer upwards from the meniscus, as a result of the differences in surface tension between the layers.

The biphasic movement is assisted by marangoni flow in helping to reform the tear film (Velarde et al., 1986). There are potentially four types of marangoni effects (i.e. effects associated with local variations in surface tension) in the tear film:

1. Tear film reformation following a blink
2. Tear film rupture
3. Mucus 'heaping' due to a temperature gradient across the tear film
4. Mucus flow at the mucus–aqueous interface, promoting mucus stabilization.

Evaporation

A small amount of tear fluid is lost passively by evaporation. Values for normal tear evaporation rates vary between research groups due to the different measuring techniques (Rolando and Refojo, 1983; Tomlinson *et al.*, 1991; Craig and Tomlinson, 1997). The more invasive the technique, the higher is the measured evaporation rate, since the tear film is being disrupted and the lipid layer can no longer inhibit evaporation of the underlying aqueous phase. No significant differences in evaporation rate have been observed between the sexes or with increasing age (Craig and Tomlinson, 1998), but tear evaporation has been found to be lowest on awakening, rising to a stable level in a short time after eye opening (Tomlinson and Giesbrecht, 1993). The lower evaporation rate is believed to be related to the altered tear chemistry, including thicker lipid and mucous layers, during eye closure (Tomlinson, 1992).

Tear evaporation has been found to increase in ocular pathological conditions where there is mucus deficiency (Refojo *et al.*, 1986), as in ocular pemphygoid or Stevens–Johnson syndrome; aqueous deficiency (Rolando *et al.*, 1983), as in keratoconjunctivitis sicca; lipid deficiency (Craig and Tomlinson, 1997), as in blepharitis or meibomian gland dysfunction (Mathers, 1993); or epithelial irregularity (Refojo *et al.*, 1986), as in scarring.

Instilling any drop onto the ocular surface disrupts the structure of the tear film and causes the rate of evaporation to increase (Trees and

Tomlinson, 1990). In the same way, all contact lenses disrupt the superficial lipid layer and cause an increase in the tear evaporation (Tomlinson and Cedarstaff, 1982). No correlation has been shown to exist between the water content of hydrogel lenses and rate of tear evaporation (Cedarstaff and Tomlinson, 1983).

Absorption

The third route for loss of lacrimal fluid is by absorption. This probably occurs from the mucosal surfaces of both the nasolacrimal duct and the conjunctiva. Values of up to 2.0 µl/min have been suggested for combined nasolacrimal and conjunctival absorption (Sørensen and Taagehøg-Jensen, 1979; Lutosky and Maurice, 1986).

Conclusion

The tear film is a dynamic structure of complex nature and function. Its components are highly interdependent and share a close relationship with the surrounding ocular tissues. Failure of a single aspect of the tear film can lead to a breakdown of the regular structure and ultimately to the symptoms and signs associated with dry eye syndrome. Attention should be paid to the use of systemic medication and contact lens status as these may be sufficient to upset the balance of components within the carefully ordered tear film structure. It is clear, from the complexity of the preocular tear film, that to facilitate more specific diagnosis and appropriate management, assessment must include evaluation of as many aspects of tear function as possible.

References

Aisen, P. and Leibman, A. (1972) Lactoferrin and transferrin: a comparative study. *Biochim. Biophys. Acta*, **257**, 314–323.

Aurell, G. and Kornerup, P. (1949) On glandular structures at the corneo-scleral junction in man and swine: the so-called 'Manz glands'. *Acta Ophthalmol.*, **27**, 19–45.

Benjamin, W. J., Piccolo, M. G. and Toubiana, H. A. (1984) Wettability: a blink by blink account. *Int. Contact Lens Clin.*, **11**, 492–498.

Bothelo, S. Y. (1964) Tears and the lacrimal gland. *Sci. Am.*, **211**, 78–86.

Bron, A. J. and Tiffany, J. M. (1998) The meibomian glands and tear film lipids; structure, function and control. *Adv. Exp. Med. Biol.*, **438**, 281–295.

Brown, S. I. and Dervichian, D. G. (1969) The oils of the meibomian glands; physical and surface characteristics. *Arch. Ophthalmol.*, **82**, 537–540.

Butcher, E. O. and Coonin, A. (1949) The physical propates of human seban. *J. Invest. Dermatol.*, **12**, 249–254.

Carney, L. G. and Hill, R. M. (1976) Human tear pH. Diurnal variations. *Arch. Ophthalmol.*, **94**, 821–824.

Cedarstaff, T. H. and Tomlinson, A. (1983) A comparative study of tear evaporation rates and water content of soft contact lenses. *Am. J. Optom. Physiol. Opt.*, **60**, 167–174.

Chung, C. W., Tigges, M. and Stone, R. A. (1996) Peptidergic innervation of the primate meibomian gland. *Invest. Ophthalmol. Vis. Sci.*, **37**, 238–245.

Craig, J. P. (1995a) Tear physiology in the normal and dry eye. PhD Thesis, Glasgow Caledonian University, pp. 63–65.

Craig, J. P. (1995b) Tear physiology in the normal and dry eye. PhD Thesis, Glasgow Caledonian University, pp. 66–72.

Craig, J. P. and Tomlinson, A. (1997) Importance of the lipid layer in human tear film stability and evaporation. *Optom. Vis. Sci.*, **74**, 8–13.

Craig, J. P. and Tomlinson, A. (1998) Age and gender effects on the normal tear film. *Adv. Exp. Med. Biol.*, **438**, 411–415.

Craig, J. P., Blades, K. and Patel, S. (1995) Tear lipid layer structure and stability following expression of the meibomian glands. *Ophthal. Physiol. Opt.*, **15**, 569–574.

Dartt, D. A. (1992) Physiology of tear production. In *The Dry Eye. A Comprehensive Guide* (eds M. A. Lemp and R. Marquardt), Berlin, Springer-Verlag, pp. 65–99.

Dartt, D. A. (1994) Regulation of tear secretion. *Adv. Exp. Med. Biol.*, **350**, 1–9.

Dilly, P. N. (1985) Contribution of the epithelium to the stability of the tear film. *Trans. Ophthalmol. Soc. UK*, **104**, 381–389.

Dilly, P. N. (1986) Subsurface vesicles and tear film mucus. In *The Preocular Tear Film in Health, Disease, and Contact Lens Wear* (ed. F. J. Holly), Lubbock, Dry Eye Institute, pp. 677–689.

Dilly, P. N. (1994) Structure and function of the tear film. *Adv. Exp. Med. Biol.*, **350**, 239–247.

Doane, M. G. (1986) Tear spreading, turnover and drainage. In *The Preocular Tear Film in Health, Disease and Contact Lens Wear* (ed. F. J. Holly), Lubbock, Dry Eye Institute, p. 659.

Doughty, M. J. (1997) Systemic drug interactions with lacrimal system, conjunctiva, cornea and lens. In *Drugs, Medications and the Eye*, Glasgow, Smawcastellane Information Services, Ch. 11.

Farris, R. L. (1985) Tear analysis in contact lens wearers. *Trans. Am. Ophthalmol. Soc.*, **83**, 501–545.

Fleiszig, S. M. J., Zaidi, T. S. and Pier, G. B. (1994) Mucus and *Pseudomonas aeruginosa* adherence to the cornea. *Adv. Exp. Med. Biol.*, **350**, 359–362.

Ford, L. C., DeLange, R. J. and Petty, R. W. (1976) Identification of a non-lysozymal bactericidal factor (beta lysin) in human tears and aqueous humor. *Am. J. Ophthalmol.*, **81**, 30–33.

Franklin, R. M., Kenyon, K. R. and Tomasi, T. B. (1973) Immunohistologic studies of human lacrimal gland: localization of immunoglobulins, secretory component and lactoferrin. *J. Immunol.*, **10**, 984–992.

Fullard, R. J. and Carney, L. G. (1984) Diurnal variation in human tear enzymes. *Exp. Eye Res.*, **38**, 15–26.

Fullard, R. J. and Carney, L. G. (1985) Human tear enzyme changes as indicators of the corneal response to anterior hypoxia. *Acta Ophthalmol.*, **63**, 678–683.

Fullard, R. J. and Carney, L. G. (1986) Use of tear enzyme activities to assess the corneal response to contact lens wear. *Acta Ophthalmol.*, **64**, 216–220.

Fullard, R. J. and Kissner, D. M. (1991) Purification of the isoforms of tear specific prealbumin. *Curr. Eye Res.*, **10**, 613–628.

Gachon, A. M., Verelle, P., Bétail, G. and Dastugue, B. (1979) Immunological and electrophoretic studies of human tear proteins. *Exp. Eye Res.*, **29**, 539–553.

Gilbard, J. P. and Kenyon, K. R. (1985) Tear diluents in the treatment of keratoconjunctivitis sicca. *Ophthalmology*, **92**, 646–650.

Gilbard, J. P., Farris, R. L. and Santamaria, J. (1978) Osmolarity of tear microvolumes in keratoconjunctivitis sicca. *Arch. Ophthalmol.*, **96**, 677–681.

Gilbard, J. P., Gray, K. L. and Rossi, S. R. (1986) A proposed mechanism for increased tear-film osmolarity in contact lens wearers. *Am. J. Ophthalmol.*, **102**, 505–507.

Gilbard, J. P., Rossi, S. R., Heyda, K. G. and Dartt, D. A. (1990) Stimulation of tear secretion by topical agents that increase cyclic nucleotide levels. *Invest. Ophthalmol. Vis. Sci.*, **31**, 1381–1388.

Glasgow, B. J., Abduragimov, A. R., Farahbakhsh, Z. *et al.* (1995) Tear lipocalins bind a broad array of lipid ligands. *Curr. Eye Res.*, **14**, 363–372.

Greiner, J. V. and Allansmith, M. R. (1981) Effect of contact lens wear on the conjunctival mucous system. *Ophthalmology*, **88**, 821–832.

Greiner, J. V., Henriquez, A. S., Weidman, T. A. *et al.* (1979) 'Second' mucous secretory system of the human conjunctiva. *Invest. Ophthalmol. Vis. Sci.*, **18(Suppl.)**, 123.

Guillon, J. P. (1986) Tear film structure in contact lenses. In *The Preocular Tear Film in Health, Disease, and Contact Lens Wear* (ed. F. J. Holly), Lubbock, Dry Eye Institute, pp. 914–939.

Guillon, J. P. (1998) Abnormal lipid layers: observation, differential diagnosis, and classification. *Adv. Exp. Med. Biol.*, **438**, 309–313.

Guillon, J. P. and Guillon, M. (1993) Tear film examination of the contact lens patient. *Optician*, **206(5421)**, 21–29.

Henderson, J. W. and Prough, W. A. (1950) Influence of age and sex on flow of tears. *Arch. Ophthalmol.*, **43**, 224–231.

Heremans, J. F. (1968) Immunoglobulin formation and function in different tissues. *Curr. Top. Microbiol. Immunol.*, **45**, 131–203.

Hill, R. M. (1984) The quantitative blink. *Int. Cont. Lens Clin.*, **11**, 366–368.

Holly, F. J. (1973) Formation and rupture of the tear film. *Exp. Eye Res.*, **15**, 515–525.

Holly, F. J. (1979) Protein and lipid absorption by acrylic hydrogels and their relationship to water wettability. *J. Polym. Sci. Polym. Symp.*, **66**, 409–417.

Holly, F. J. (1981a) Tear film physiology and contact lens wear: I. Pertinent aspects of tear film physiology. *Am. J. Optom. Physiol. Opt.*, **58**, 324–330.

Holly, F. J. (1981b) Tear film physiology and contact lens wear: II. Contact lens tear film interaction. *Am. J. Optom. Physiol. Opt.*, **58**, 331–341.

Holly, F. J. and Lamberts, D. W. (1981) Effect of non-isotonic solutions on tear film osmolarity. *Invest. Ophthalmol. Vis. Sci.*, **20**, 236–245.

Holly, F. J. and Lemp, M. A. (1971) Wettability and wetting of corneal epithelium. *Exp. Eye Res.*, **11**, 239–250.

Holly, F. J. and Lemp, M. A. (1977) Tear physiology and dry eyes. *Surv. Ophthalmol.*, **22**, 69–87.

Iwata, S., Lemp, M. A., Holly, F. J. and Dohlman, C. H. (1969) Evaporation rate of water from the precorneal tear film and cornea in the rabbit. *Invest. Ophthalmol.*, **8**, 613–619.

Janssen, P. T. and van Bjisterveld, O. P. (1983) Origin and biosynthesis of human tear fluid proteins. *Invest. Ophthalmol. Vis. Sci.*, **24**, 623–630.

Jaseplson, A. S. and Lockwood, A. W. (1964) Immunoelectrophoretic studies of the protein components of normal tears. *J. Immunol.*, **93**, 532–539.

Jordan, A. and Baum, J. (1980) Basic tear flow. Does it exist? *Ophthalmology*, **87**, 920–930.

Kaura, R. and Tiffany, J. M. (1986) The role of mucous glycoproteins. In *The Preocular Tear Film in Health, Disease, and Contact Lens Wear* (ed. F. J. Holly), Lubbock, Dry Eye Institute, pp. 728–732.

Kessing, S. V. (1968) Mucous gland system of the conjunctiva. *Acta Ophthalmol.*, **95(Suppl.)**, 1–133.

Kessler, T. L. and Dartt, D. A. (1994) Neural stimulation of conjunctival goblet cell mucus secretion in rats. *Adv. Exp. Med. Biol.*, **350**, 393–398.

Kilp, H. (1978) Biochemistry. In *Soft Contact Lenses, Clinical, and Applied Technology* (ed. M. Ruben), New York, John Wiley and Sons, pp. 117–142.

King-Smith, P. E., Fogt, N., Fink, B. A. *et al.* (1998) A tear layer thickness of 1.6 to 7.3 μm determined from reflectance spectra. *Invest. Ophthalmol. Vis. Sci.*, **39**, S533.

King-Smith, P. E., Fink, B. A. and Fogt, N. (1999) Three interferometric methods for measuring the thickness of layers of the tear film. *Optom. Vis. Sci.*, **76**, 19–32.

Kwok, L. S. (1984) Calculation and application of the anterior surface area of a human model cornea. *Theor. Biol.*, **108**, 295–313.

Lin, S. P. and Brenner, H. (1986) Stability of the tear film. In *The Preocular Tear Film in Health, Disease, and Contact Lens Wear* (ed. F. J. Holly), Lubbock, Dry Eye Institute, pp. 670–676.

Liotet, S., van Bijsterveld, O. P., Kogbe, O. and Laroche, L. (1987) A new hypothesis on tear film stability. *Ophthalmologica*, **195**, 119–124.

Lowther, G. E. (1997) Handling hydrogel lens patients with contact lens tear-film problems. In *Dryness, Tears and Contact Lens Wear* (eds G. E. Lowther and C. D. Leahy), Oxford, Butterworth-Heinemann, pp. 54–83.

Lutosky, S. and Maurice, D. M. (1986) Absorption of tears by the nasolacrimal system. In *The Preocular Tear Film in Health, Disease, and Contact Lens Wear* (ed. F. J. Holly), Lubbock, Dry Eye Institute, pp. 663–669.

Manz, G. (1859) Über neue eugentumliche drusen um cornealrande und über den bau des limbus conjunctivae. *Zschr. F. Rat Med.*, **3(Suppl.)**, 22–28.

Mathers, W. D. (1993) Ocular evaporation in meibomian gland dysfunction and dry eye. *Ophthalmology*, **100**, 347–351.

McClellan, B. H., Whitney, C. R., Newman, L. P. *et al.* (1973) Immunoglobulins in the tears. *Am. J. Ophthalmol.*, **76**, 89–101.

McCulley, J. P. and Sciallis, G. F. (1977) Meibomian keratoconjunctivitis. *Am. J. Ophthalmol.*, **84**, 788–793.

McDonald, J. E. (1968) Surface phenomena of tear films. *Trans. Am. Ophthalmol. Soc.*, **66,** 905–909.

Milder, B. (1987) The lacrimal apparatus. In *Adler's Physiology of the Eye*, 8th edn (eds R. A. Moses and W. M. Hart), St Louis, Mosby, pp. 15–35.

Mishima. S. (1965) Some physiological aspects of the precorneal tear film. *Arch. Ophthalmol.*, **73,** 233–241.

Mishima, S. and Maurice, D. M. (1961) The oily layer of the tear film and evaporation from the corneal surface. *Exp. Eye Res.*, **1,** 39–45.

Mishima, S., Gasset, A., Klyce, S. D. and Baum, J. L. (1966) Determination of tear volume and tear flow. *Invest. Ophthalmol.*, **5,** 264–276.

Neutra, M. R. and LeBlond, C. P. (1966) Synthesis of the carbohydrate of mucus in the golgi complex as shown by electron microscope radio-autography of goblet cells from rats injected with glucose-H3. *J. Cell Biol.*, **30,** 119–136.

Norn, M. S. (1966) The conjunctival fluid. Its height, volume, density of cells, and flow. *Acta Ophthalmol.*, **44,** 212–222.

Norn, M. S. (1969a) Desiccation of the precorneal film. I. Corneal wetting time. *Acta Ophthalmol.*, **47,** 865–880.

Norn, M. S. (1969b) Dead, degenerate and living cells in conjunctival fluid and mucous thread. *Acta Ophthalmol.*, **47,** 1102–1115.

Norn, M. S. (1979) Semiquantitative interference study of the fatty layer of precorneal tear film. *Acta Ophthalmol.*, **57,** 766–774.

O'Leary, D. J. and Wilson, G. (1993) *Transactions of the ISCLR Meeting*, Hayman Islands, Australia.

Perra, M. T., Latini, M. S., Serra, A. *et al.* (1990) A histochemical study for androgen metabolic enzymes. *Invest. Ophthalmol. Vis. Sci.*, **31,** 771–773.

Perra, M. T., Serra, A., Sirigu, P. and Turno, F. (1996) Histochemical demonstration of acetylcholinesterase activity in human meibomian glands. *Eur. J. Histochem.*, **40,** 39–44.

Port, M. J. A. and Asaria, T. S. (1990) The assessment of tear volume. *J. Br. Cont. Lens Assoc.*, **13,** 76–82.

Prydal, J. I., Artal, P., Woon, H. and Campbell, F. W. (1992) Study of the human precorneal tear film thickness and structure using laser interferometry. *Invest. Ophthalmol. Vis. Sci.*, **33,** 2006–2011.

Prydal, J. I., Kerr-Muir, M. G. and Dilly, P. N. (1993) Comparison of tear thickness in three species determined by the glass fibre method and confocal microscopy. *Eye*, **7,** 472–475.

Puffer, M. J., Neault, R. W. and Brubacker, R. F. (1980) Basal precorneal tear turnover in the human eye. *Am. J. Ophthalmol.*, **89,** 369–376.

Records, R. E. (1979) Tear film. In *Physiology of the Eye and Visual System* (ed. R. E. Records), Hagerstown, Harper & Row, pp. 47–67.

Redl, B., Holzfeind, P. and Lottspeicht, F. (1992) cDNA cloning and sequencing reveals human tear prealbumin to be a member of the lipophilic-ligand carrier protein superfamily. *J. Biol. Chem.*, **267,** 20282–20287.

Refojo, M. F., Rolando, M., Belldegrün, R. and Kenyon, K. R. (1986) Tear evaporimeter for diagnosis and research. In *The Preocular Tear Film in Health, Disease, and Contact Lens Wear* (ed. F. J. Holly), Lubbock, Dry Eye Institute, pp. 117–126.

Rohen, J. W. and Lütjen-Drecoll, E. (1992) Functional morphology or the conjunctiva. In *The Dry Eye. A Comprehensive Guide* (eds M. A. Lemp and R. Marquardt), Berlin, Springer-Verlag, pp. 35–63.

Rolando, M. and Refojo, M. F. (1983) Tear evaporimeter for measuring water evaporation from the tear film under controlled conditions in humans. *Exp. Eye Res.*, **36**, 25–33.

Rolando, M., Refojo, M. F. and Kenyon, K. R. (1983) Increased tear evaporation in eyes with keratoconjunctivitis sicca. *Arch. Ophthalmol.*, **101**, 557–558.

Ruskell, G. L. (1985) Innervation of the conjunctiva. *Trans. Ophthalmol. Soc. UK*, **104**, 390–395.

Sapse, A. T., Bonavida, B., Stone, W. Jr. and Sercarz, E. E. (1969) Proteins in human tears. I. Immunoelectrophoretic patterns. *Arch. Ophthalmol.*, **81**, 815–819.

Schoenwald, R. D., Vidvauns, S., Wurster, D. E. and Barfknecht, C. F. (1998) The role of tear proteins in tear film stability in the dry eye patient and in the rabbit. *Adv. Exp. Med. Biol.*, **438**, 391–400.

Seal, D. V., McGill, J. I., Mackie, I. A. *et al.* (1986) Bacteriology and tear protein profiles of the dry eye. *Br. J. Ophthalmol.*, **70**, 122–125.

Sharma, A. and Ruckenstein, E. (1985) Mechanism of tear film rupture and its implications for contact lens tolerance. *Am. J. Optom. Physiol. Opt.*, **62**, 246–253.

Sirigu, P., Shen, R. L. and Pinto da Silva, P. (1992) Human meibomian glands: the ultrastructure of acinar cells as viewed by thin section and freeze-fracture transmission electron microscopies. *Invest. Ophthalmol. Vis. Sci.*, **33**, 2284–2292.

Sørensen, T. and Taagehøg Jensen, F. (1979) Conjunctival transport of technetium-99m pertechnetate. *Acta Ophthalmol.*, **57**, 691–699.

Takakusaki, I. (1969) Fine structure of the human palpebral conjunctiva with special reference to pathological changes in vernal conjunctivitis. *Arch. Histol. Japan*, **30**, 247–282.

Temel, A., Kazokoglu, H., Taga, Y. *et al.* (1991) The effect of contact lens wear on tear immunoglobulins. *CLAO. J.*, **17**, 69–71.

Terry, J. E. and Hill, R. M. (1978) Human tear osmotic pressure. Diurnal variations and the closed eye. *Arch. Ophthalmol.*, **96**, 120–122.

Thody, A. J. and Shuster, S. (1979) Control and function of sebaceous glands. *Physiol. Rev.*, **2**, 383–416.

Tiffany, J. M. (1978) Individual variations in human meibomian lipid composition. *Exp. Eye Res.*, **27**, 289–300.

Tiffany, J. M. (1987) The lipid secretion of the meibomian glands. *Adv. Lipid Res.*, **22**, 1–62.

Tiffany, J. M. (1988) Tear film stability and contact lens wear. *J. Br. Cont. Lens Assoc.*, **11**, 35–38.

Tiffany, J. M. (1990a) Measurement of wettability of the corneal epithelium. I. Particle attachment method. *Acta Ophthalmol.*, **68**, 175–181.

Tiffany, J. M. (1990b) Measurement of wettability of the corneal epithelium. II. Contact angle method. *Acta Ophthalmol.*, **68**, 182–187.

Tiffany, J. M. (1994) Composition and biophysical properties of the tear film: knowledge and uncertainty. *Adv. Exp. Med. Biol.*, **350**, 231–238.

Tiffany, J. M. and Marsden, R. G. (1986) The influence of composition on physical properties of meibomian secretion. In *The Preocular Tear Film in Health, Disease, and Contact Lens Wear* (ed. F. J. Holly), Lubbock, Dry Eye Institute, pp. 597–608.

Tomlinson, A. (1992) Tear film changes with contact lens wear. In *Complications of Contact Lens Wear* (ed. A. Tomlinson), St Louis, Mosby, pp. 159–194.

Tomlinson, A. and Cedarstaff, T. H. (1982) Tear evaporation from the human eye. The effects of contact lens wear. *J. Br. Cont. Lens Assoc.*, **5**, 141–150.

Tomlinson, A. and Giesbrecht, C. (1993) The ageing tear film. *J. Br. Cont. Lens Assoc.*, **16**, 67–69.

Tomlinson, A., Trees, G. R. and Occhipinti, J. R. (1991) Tear production and evaporation in the normal eye. *Ophthal. Physiol. Opt.*, **11**, 44–47.

Trees, G. R. and Tomlinson, A. (1990) Effect of artificial tear solutions and saline on tear film evaporation. *Optom. Vis. Sci.*, **67**, 886–890.

van Haeringen, N. J. and Glasius, E. (1974) Enzymatic studies in lacrimal secretion. *Exp. Eye Res.*, **19**, 135–139.

Velarde, M. G., Murube del Castillo, J., Castillo, J. L. and García, M. (1986) Marangoni-Bénard convection and macrodynamics of tear film flow. In *The Preocular Tear Film in Health, Disease, and Contact Lens Wear* (ed. F. J. Holly), Lubbock, Dry Eye Institute, pp. 688–696.

Versura, P., Maltarello, M. C., Cellini, M. *et al.* (1986) Detection of mucus glycoconjugates in human conjunctiva by using the lectin-colloid gold technique in TEM. II. A quantitative study in dry eye patients. *Acta Ophthalmol.*, **64**, 451–455.

Wanko, T., Lloyd, B. J. and Mathews, J. (1964) The fine structure of the human conjunctiva in the perlimbal zone. *Invest. Ophthalmol.*, **3**, 285–301.

Wolff, E. (1946) Muco-cutaneous junction of the lid margin and the distribution of tear fluid. *Trans. Ophthalmol. Soc. UK*, **66**, 291–308.

Wright, P. (1985) Normal tear production and drainage. *Trans. Ophthalmol. Soc. UK*, **104**, 351–354.

Yamada, M., Mochizuki, H., Kawai, M. *et al.* (1997) Fluorophotometric measurement of pH of human tears in vivo. *Curr. Eye Res.*, **16**, 482–486.

3 Current clinical techniques to study the tear film and tear secretions

Jean-Pierre Guillon

Introduction

The occurrence of dry eye symptoms is so common that the detection and differentiation of tear film abnormalities is the concern of every clinician. The definition of an abnormal tear film and its causes have been reviewed by many authors (Holly and Lemp, 1977; Bron, 1985; Lemp 1995), who consider the following signs to be important when diagnosing the condition:

- A scanty or uneven meniscus
- The presence of excessive particulate matter
- The rupture of the tear film prior to a subsequent blink
- The production of hyperosmotic tears
- The abnormality or absence of the superficial lipid layer
- An abnormal or inadequate mucous layer
- The presence of an epithelial surface disorder.

The factors leading to the production of an abnormal tear film are numerous and include the following:

- Insufficient lacrimation
- Increased evaporation and a low tear turnover rate
- Increased polarity of the meibomian secretion
- Abnormal tear protein composition
- Inadequate blink behaviour
- Inadequate mucus supply and mucous layer
- A primary ocular surface disorder.

Some of these signs can be detected as a matter of routine clinical observation using non-invasive techniques or with simple tests available to the practitioner. A large number of clinical, experimental, and research techniques have been developed to study the tear film and its different components. This chapter provides an overview of the relevant techniques that can be applied by clinicians who wish to improve their examination of the tear film and the detection of dry eye.

Any detection routine must start with the assessment of symptoms and the use of a battery of tests that permit the clinician to determine the type of tear problem present and its origin (lipid, aqueous, mucous, surface anomaly or multiple causes), and grade the severity of damage to the ocular surface. The goal of the evaluation is to choose the most relevant and effective therapy for the individual subject.

Patient history and subjective symptoms

The presence and nature of symptoms needs to be ascertained before any examination, and their presence and status must be monitored to evaluate the effect of any treatment given. Symptoms vary in type and severity according to the state of instability of the tear film and the resultant damage to the ocular surface. These symptoms and their causes include:

- In marginal cases, a sensation of burning may be caused by the hypertonic shift in the tear film
- Tearing may also be present as a reflex and protective mechanism, induced by external conditions of low relative humidity, smog or air conditioning, and associated with the break-up of the tear film
- Poor lubrication at night or incomplete lid closure may result in difficulty in opening the eyes on awakening
- Mucous discharge may indicate instability of the mucous layer and its dehydration
- Foreign-body sensations may be caused by improper lubrication and should be a warning of the possibility of more severe tear film conditions
- Dryness may be recognized as a sensation and reported as dry, scratchy, gritty or sandy
- Photophobia may occur in the presence of continuing irritation
- Blurred vision may be the result of a non-wetting ocular surface in Sjögren's disease and keratoconjunctivitis sicca
- Pain will be reported when deep epithelial damage is present.

The use of a patient questionnaire is beneficial as it allows the grading of symptoms and is repeatable for comparison purposes before, during and after treatment. Many questionnaires exist; the one most commonly used by optometrists for screening purposes is the McMonnies questionnaire

(McMonnies, 1986; McMonnies and Ho, 1986, 1987a, 1987b). Other questionnaires have been developed to include more specific questions relating to contact lens wear (Robboy and Osborn, 1988; Guillon *et al.*, 1992) or for use as a predictive and diagnostic tool in clinical research (Fullard and Snyder, 1995). In these questionnaires, a value is assigned to each question and the total score obtained is an indication of the presence and severity of the symptoms.

Rolando *et al.* (1997) have separated the questionnaire into six sections:

1. Fundamental symptoms
2. Accessory symptoms
3. Environmental stress conditions
4. Need for topical therapy
5. Use of systemic drugs
6. Presence of systemic diseases.

This comprehensive analysis can provide a reasonable understanding of the origin of ocular surface disease, but a quantitative scoring will give more precise information on the level of risk that the patient faces from a tear film related ocular surface disease. Dry eye questionnaires have also been designed and used for large population studies of the prevalence of reported symptoms (Doughty *et al.*, 1997). These questionnaires allow the clinician to choose the spectrum and depth of information to suit the particular needs of general screening or detailed evaluation of symptoms.

Biomicroscopic examination

The routine biomicroscopic examination provides invaluable information and allows the following tests to be carried out:

- Assessment of the appearance of the tear meniscus
- Observation of superficial particulate movement
- Observation of surface interference phenomena either by simple specular reflection or with the Tearscope Plus™ (Keeler Instruments, Broomall, PA)
- Measurement of non-invasive break-up time (NIBUT)
- Use of vital dyes (fluorescein, rose bengal and lissamine green) to allow the study of the health of the ocular surface and its response to treatment
- Examination of the lid borders, the lashes and related glands for any signs of blockage, abnormality or pathology

- Examination of the meibomian glands when the lower lid is pulled down, using transillumination with a simple light source through the palpebral conjunctiva
- Detection of lid pathology, such as blepharitis, as well as age-related degenerative changes to the gland orifices or the lid borders
- Assessment of localized conjunctival hyperaemia, preferably using grading scales for increased precision and repeatability
- Observation of the blink movement.

Observations of the tear meniscus

The total tear volume found within the palpebral aperture has been estimated at between 7 µl and 10 µl (Maurice, 1973). Up to 90 per cent of the tear volume is found in the superior and inferior marginal tear strip, also known as the (lid) tear meniscus. Norn (1965) found that 75 per cent of the total volume of preocular tear fluid is in the meniscus and 25 per cent in the preocular tear film (POTF). An extra 20–30 µl can be held between the lids if care is taken to avoid blinking. When blinking is permitted, any amount above 10 µl will be flushed out of a normal palpebral fissure (Maurice, 1973), although the amount will vary with the size of the palpebral fissure.

It also appears that there is very little fluid in the fornices. For example, if the lower lid is pulled away from the surface of the eye, some tear fluid will invade the newly created space. But when the lid is released, the tear fluid is expelled by apposition to reform the marginal tear strip. No tear reserve is present at the inner canthus, which is only moist.

The tear reservoir or meniscus forms along the lower and upper lid. Each meniscus is limited on the lid margin side by the muco-cutaneous junction (line of Marx) situated just behind the meibomian gland orifices. On the corneal side, the meniscus is separated from the POTF by a localized thinning known as the 'black line', which is only visible when the film is stained with fluorescein (Holly, 1978). The 'black line' separates the POTF from the marginal tear strips and represents an area of thinning of the tear film (McDonald and Brubaker, 1971). Examination of the 'black line' has shown that there is no diffusion of dye across the line, and when fluid accumulates in the lower marginal strip the line moves away from the lid margin (Maurice, 1980).

The formation of the tear meniscus depends on the balance between the negative pressure induced by its concave surface and the hydrostatic pressure due to the height of the fluid column in the meniscus (Holly, 1980). In the presence of a restricted amount of fluid (as in the ocular environment) an imbalance is created because the tear film cannot replenish the aspirated fluid fast enough by interlaminal flow (Holly,

1980). The aspiration is the result of an unsaturated or 'thirsty' meniscus and leads to localized thinning of the film (McDonald and Brubaker, 1971). Slit-lamp observation of the 'black line' and of the curvature of the meniscus gives some information as to the degree to which the meniscus is unsaturated. The smaller the radius of curvature the more 'thirsty' the meniscus; hence, when the meniscus gets larger and less curved, it becomes less 'thirsty' as a larger volume of fluid is available (Holly, 1980).

The observation of lid meniscus height (Baum, 1973) and its irregularity (Rolando *et al.*, 1990) has been proposed as a guide to the diagnosis of dry eye. The lower meniscus is easier to examine for regularity, height, width and curvature. Holly and Lemp (1977) estimated its width to be approximately 1 mm and suggested that a scanty appearance or area of discontinuity were signs of an aqueous tear deficiency or lipid abnormality. Taylor (1980) suggested that the meniscus should be described qualitatively as intact, non-intact or temporally non-intact. Although several authors (Klein, 1949; Wright, 1971; Baum, 1973) have proposed the evaluation of the tear meniscus as an assessment of tear flow, Lamberts *et al.* (1979) found that the tear meniscus height in normal eyes varied between 0.3 mm and 0.1 mm in 92 per cent of his 86 observations, and that there was no correlation between tear meniscus height and Schirmer test result with and without anaesthesia.

Terry (1984) concluded that a tear meniscus height < 0.3 mm was an indication of dry eye. Port and Asaria (1990) modified a corneal pachometer to carry out accurate measurements of tear prism height. However, these authors obtained the lowest values of all investigators and it is thought that this was due to the relative drying of the tear prism by the slit-lamp light.

Meniscus morphology

The reflection of a light beam moved vertically across the tear meniscus gives an assessment of its curvature (McDonald, 1969). The normal meniscus should have a convex surface near the corneal side, a concave surface centrally and a convex curve in its contact with the eyelids.

A scanty or uneven meniscus is seen as an irregular reflection originating from its very small curvature bordering the lid edge when using direct illumination. An uneven border line and a height < 0.1 mm, combined with a sharp definition of the 'black line' separating it from the tear film, are signs of abnormality. Localized tear film break-up originating from the meniscus border is increased in these cases. An increased curvature is a sign of reduced volume but also of reduced hydrostatic pressure; the reduction in pressure encourages movement of fluid from the POTF and the meniscus, inducing localized disruption. The shape of the meniscus can be observed in the specular reflection zone of the biomicroscope as a bright central band bordered by dark, non-reflective areas.

The Tearscope Plus™ illuminates the tear meniscus along its whole length and permits the non-invasive observation of morphological changes during the blink sequence. In the central area of observation, the tear meniscus presents a black central band bordered by bright bands on the lid side and the tear film side (Figure 3.1). Any irregularity of the meniscus shape caused by degenerative lid changes or meibomian gland blockage can be seen as a distortion of the central black band. Any variation in tear meniscus height can also be observed along its length (Figure 3.2). With practice, the clinician can readily grade the appearance and height of the tear meniscus using this instrument.

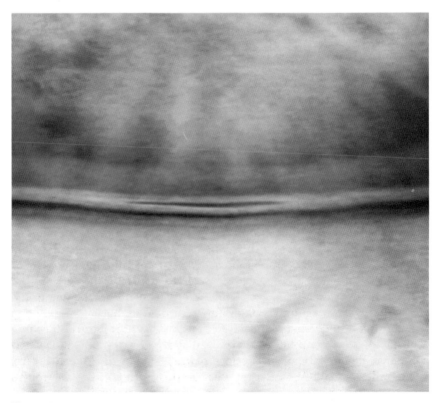

Figure 3.1

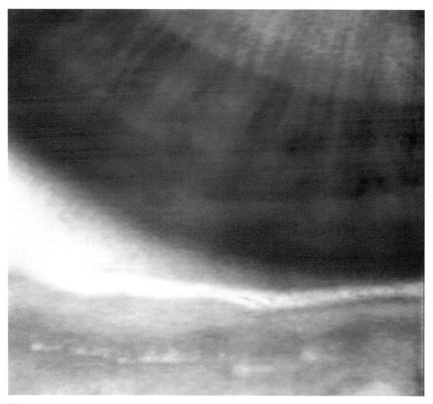

Figure 3.2

Conjunctival signs

It has been suggested that the presence of 'lip-like folds of the inferior conjunctiva' is a sign of tear film related ocular surface problems. They categorized these folds into three grades: in grade 1 the folds are barely visible in the temporal corner; in grade 2 they are clearly visible in the temporal bulbar conjunctiva; and in grade 3 they are also visible in the conjunctiva corresponding to the inferior corneal limbus.

Hoh *et al.* (1995) described the presence of lid-parallel conjunctival folds (LIPCOF) bordering the posterior lid margin in dry eye patients and compared their predictive value to a battery of tests of ocular dryness. Four grades of LIPCOF were proposed: grade 0 with no permanent folds in the primary position; grade 1 where individual small folds in the primary position appear lower than the normal tear meniscus; grade 2 where multiple folds usually appear in the primary position up to the height of normal tear film meniscus; and grade 3 where multiple folds usually appear in primary position higher than normal tear film meniscus. In dry eye, the LIPCOF has a negative predictive value of 76 per cent and a positive predictive value of 93 per cent. Grade 1 subjects have a 15-fold higher risk of having dry eye compared to grade 0. For grades 2 and 3 the risk factor is 63 times and 190 times higher respectively.

Although the authors do not explain the mechanism involved, it seems that the folds disturb the morphology of the meniscus and its relationship with the lid edge. In the presence of folds the reservoir morphology is abnormal, thus limiting the uptake of tears during the blink and reducing the resurfacing of the POTF over the conjunctival surface. Further alterations to the conjunctival surface may occur and increase the signs and symptoms of dry eye.

Particulate matter

The presence of excessive particulate matter in the POTF and meniscus, when viewed with either high and low magnification, is abnormal. This particulate matter often consists of mucous strands of increased length formed by mucus dislodged from the epithelial surface and mixed with the superficial lipid layer. In filamentary keratitis these strands will be strongly attached to the surface epithelial cells.

Increased cellular debris is indicative of surface damage when observed in contact lens wear or in conjunction with the use of preservatives and in response to conjunctival inflammation (Bron, 1985). Keratoconjunctivitis sicca (KCS) patients exhibit a quantifiable increase in cellular debris in the tear film following rapid desquamation of damaged cells (Bron, 1985).

McDonald (1969) evaluated the speed of movement of the tear film by observing the movement of particles found at its surface, such as mucous strands, dust, air or lipid bubbles, or desquamated cells. These observations allow the classification of the viscosity of the tears as the inverse of the speed of flow of particles. A reduced viscosity will be associated with a fast movement of particles and a high viscosity with a slow movement of particles. Practice and numerous observations will be necessary to assess the normal velocity and the related subjective measurement of viscosity.

Schuller et al. (1972) and Hill (1981) found a good correlation between this method and tear viscosity measurements. Hill (1981) suggested that the viscosity rating tests could help in identifying the prospective wearer prone to contact lens deposition.

Observation of interference phenomena

Surface phenomena of the tear film have been observed since the slit-lamp biomicroscope was first developed. Yet only over the past few years has photography of these phenomena been possible. Following the work of early pioneers, the study of interference phenomena was advanced by Ehlers (1965). In his extensive dissertation, Ehlers described the biomicroscopic examination of the precorneal film, the presence of embedded particles and various colour dispersion phenomena visible in the portion lying slightly outside the direct 'mirror zone' formed by the light reflected from the cornea. He concluded that these phenomena could be due to small droplets of secretions discharged from the meibomian glands.

McDonald (1969) studied the surface phenomena of the tear film on the eye, on contact lenses, in humans and in the rabbit. He used the biomicroscope to observe the reflection of a fluorescent light or gooseneck lamp placed close to the cornea to produce spectral interference patterns visible in front of the virtual image of the lamp. McDonald concluded that the grey background observed corresponded to a surface layer not thick enough to cause interference ($< 1000\,\text{Å}$). The first order of spectrum of interference was present for thicknesses from $1000–1750\,\text{Å}$ and a second order spectrum of colours corresponded to a layer thickness of $1750–5200\,\text{Å}$. He suggested that the interference patterns were confined to the oily layer and interpreted fractures in this layer as indicating a breakdown of its viscosity.

Using theoretical analysis and reflectometry measurement, Clark and Carney (1971) showed that most of the reflection originates from the oily layer present at the anterior surface of the film. Clark (1973) used interferometry techniques to measure the anterior surface topography and thickness variation of the precorneal tear film.

Norn (1979) devised a semi-quantitative method of measuring the lipid layer by observation of the specular reflex. In this method, if a red petrol-like pattern appears on the precorneal tear film when the eyes are fully opened, the lipid layer must be no less than 134 nm thick; if the specular reflection is colourless or presents greyish lines, the lipid layer is thinner. The patient is asked to close the eye until the interference colours appear. The lipid layer becomes thicker in response to gradual narrowing of the palpebral aperture. For example, if the palpebral aperture size has to be halved to produce interference colours, the lipid layer thickness can be calculated as at least $134\,\text{nm} \times 0.5 = 67\,\text{nm}$. This technique may be used clinically, but the calculations used, the variability in measurement and the irregular nature of the lipid layer will limit its precision.

Norn examined 206 normal subjects and found an average lipid layer thickness of $102 \pm 3\,\text{nm}$. Only 5 per cent showed a maximum layer ($\geq 200\,\text{nm}$) and 8 per cent a minimum layer ($\geq 17\,\text{nm}$, corresponding to a palpebral fissure ≥2 mm). A maximum thickness was noted on awakening, took 20–60 minutes to stabilize and was independent of age, sex and break-up time (BUT). An increased thickness was found in chronic blepharitis (129 ± 8 nm), in acute infectious conjunctivitis (164 ± 7 nm), and with all conditions complicated by bacterial infection.

Other authors have described various microscopy techniques for observing interference phenomena. Hamano *et al.* (1980a) used a biodifferential interference microscope on normal rabbit and human tear films, and also in cases of palpebral entropion, trichiasis, superficial keratitis, corneal erosion, corneal ulcer, epithelial desquamation and Sjögren's syndrome. Guillon (1982) described his technique of high magnification observations of tear film layers under polarized light with photographs of irregular lipid layer and dust particles at the surface of the POTF. Kilp *et al.* (1982) used a reflecting microscope at high magnification and also differential interference contrast microscopy to study the surface irregularities of the tear film. Josephson (1983) described a technique for the observation of the lipid layer of the POTF over the bulbar conjunctiva near the temporal border of the limbus. Lydon and Guillon (1984) used a wide field technique in the photography of the lipid layer of the POTF at 1:1 or 2:1 magnification. Knoll and Walters (1985) employed a modified Bausch & Lomb keratometer to

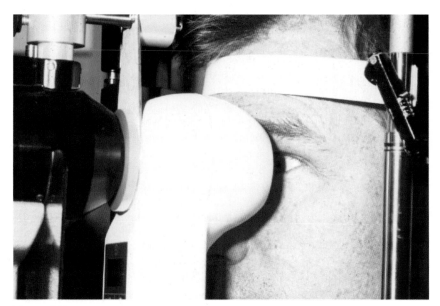

Figure 3.3

photograph the changes in the specular reflection from the anterior surface of the tear film formed on rigid gas-permeable and hydrogel lenses. Olsen (1985) used a slit-lamp photometer to measure the reflectivity of the corneal reflex. His findings are consistent with a 40 nm thick oily layer.

Since the development of the Tearscope (Guillon, 1986; Figure 3.3), Jean-Pierre Guillon has proposed a classification of the appearance of the lipid layer at the surface of the POTF and of the prelens tear film (PLTF) for both soft and rigid lenses (Guillon, 1990). Five main categories of normal lipid appearance are graded in order of increasing thickness and visibility: open meshwork, tight meshwork, waves (Figure 3.4), amorphous and colours (of the first order of interference; Figure 3.5). The abnormal appearances of the layer are described as globular, abnormal colours (second or third order of interference) and lipid break-up. Their distribution in the normal population has been reported along with non-invasive measurement of their break-up time (Guillon and Guillon, 1994).

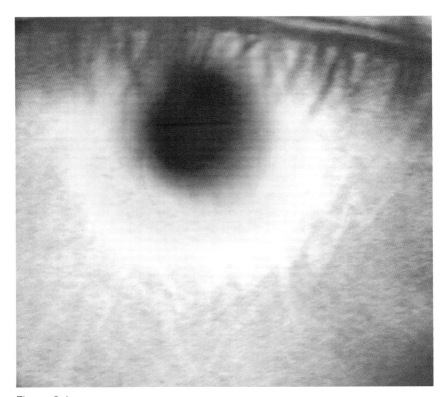

Figure 3.4

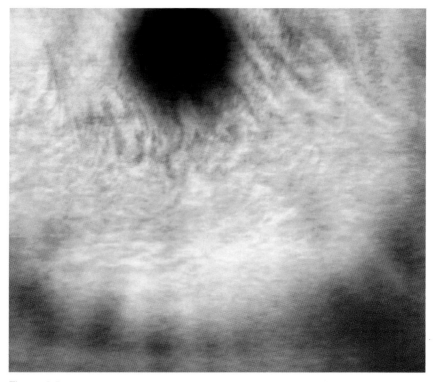

Figure 3.5

Jean-Pierre and Michel Guillon have used the techniques of wide field specular reflection for the observation of the lipid layer in numerous studies (Guillon and Guillon, 1988a, 1988b, 1988c), and have shown the importance of the lipid layer for the protection of the ocular structure in contact lens wear (Guillon *et al.*, 1989, 1991, 1992).

Recently, Craig and Tomlinson (1997) have demonstrated a link between the lipid layer, evaporation and tear film stability in humans. They found that when the human lipid layer is absent or is not confluent, and the tear film is unstable, tear evaporation is increased four-fold. They also confirmed that NIBUT varies significantly with the lipid layer appearance and that the poorest stability occurs with absent or abnormal colour fringe patterns. Korb *et al.* (1997) recently reviewed the importance of the lipid layer in contact lens wear. The abnormality or absence of the superficial lipid layer or its contamination has been observed repeatedly since McDonald (1968) first introduced the concept (Hamano *et al.*, 1980b; Guillon, 1982; Josephson, 1983).

Abnormality of the lipid layer is caused by:

- An abnormal blockage of the secretion ducts – Norn (1985) stated that: 'the orifice is sometimes blocked (in an average of 55 per cent of the glands in normals), in some cases by epithelial plugs'
- Poor apposition of the lid margin or an abnormal position of the strand orifices
- Contamination by skin lipid and/or make-up and skin lotions
- The presence of blepharitis or facial skin disorders
- Contamination by excessive or denatured mucous discharge.

Destabilization of the tear film also occurs with changes in lipid composition. An increase in free fatty acids or triglycerides, or an abnormal ratio of its polar and non-polar components, may alter and destabilize the lipid film formation. The presence of a meibomianitis has been also associated with aqueous deficiency in some cases (McCulley and Sciallis, 1977). An abnormal or inadequate mucous layer contains coarse hydrophobic strands of mucus accumulated when the mucus supply cannot keep up with accelerated mucus loss induced by increased lipid contamination, disrupted mucus-lysozyme interaction (Lee *et al.*, 1981) or increased exfoliation of surface cells.

Break-up time measurement

The POTF in humans does not remain stable for long periods of time (Holly, 1981). When blinking is prevented, the tear film ruptures within 15–40 s, dry spots appear over the cornea (Lemp and Hamill, 1973) and the tear film decreases in thickness by around 10 per cent through evaporation. A lipid film is seldom stable for long periods of time; some of the superficial lipids will migrate to the epithelium interface, contaminating the adsorbed mucin layer, creating areas of high interfacial tension and converting it into a hydrophobic surface. This process will be accelerated by local thinning of the tear film induced by the surface tension gradients in the superficial lipid layer, or by gross irregularity in the epithelial surface. The tear film in these areas becomes unstable, forming non-wettable areas of gradually increasing size.

Observation of the rupture of the POTF before a subsequent blink is the most commonly used test of tear film stability. Reduced tear film break-up time or limited ocular surface wetting measured with or without fluorescein instillation is one of the main signs of an abnormal tear film. The tear film break-up time test was proposed by Norn (1969) as corneal wetting time. A moistened fluorescein strip is applied to the bulbar conjunctiva and, after two or three blinks to spread the fluorescein evenly, the tear film is viewed with the help of a blue filter in front of the illumination system of the slit-lamp biomicroscope. When a dark area appears in the uniform coloration, it represents the rupture of the tear film and the time elapsed since the last blink is recorded as break-up time (BUT).

Norn (1969) found a mean BUT value of 30 s, but a large coefficient of variation (31 per cent) which was also reported by Vanley *et al.* (1977). Forst (1976) showed the need for repeated measurements although this is disputed by Lemp and Hamill (1973) and Rengstorff (1974). A BUT of < 10 s usually reveals an anomaly of the POTF. If the film ruptures repeatedly in the same area, a superficial epithelial abnormality must be suspected (Lemp *et al.*, 1970). If the rupture occurs near the meniscus, the thinning induced by its proximity might be the cause (McDonald and Brubaker, 1971); alternatively, partial or incomplete blinking will result in break-up over the inferior part of the ocular surface.

Variation in measurements of break-up time

Many factors affect the measurement of BUT. Those reducing the BUT include the use of local anaesthetic, exposure to benzalkonium chloride (BAK) as a preservative agent, the use of certain ointments, the presence of air convection during testing, forced blinking before measurement or holding the lids forcibly open during measurement. Those increasing the BUT are the instillation of mucomimetics (Holly, 1978) and other eye drops enhancing tear film stability, and a decrease in fluorescein concentration, the optimum value for which has been reported to be 0.5 per cent (Forst, 1978).

In fact, various concentrations and volumes of fluorescein have been suggested; Norn (1983) used 10 µl of 0.125 per cent, Forst (1978) 0.5 per cent and Stodtmeister *et al.* (1983) 1 µl of 5 per cent fluorescein. The main problem with BUT measurement is its invasive nature. When used in a routine clinical situation, involving moist impregnated strips, too many variables remain uncontrolled. Variations in the concentration and pH of the fluorescein solution, the size of the instilled drops, and the presence of preservative are probably the main sources of error.

Fluorescein dyes the aqueous phase of the tear film and has little effect on the lipid or mucous layers. In view of the finite size of the aqueous phase it seems that a minimal amount of unpreserved dye, in an adequate concentration and instilled in a precise volume, will improve the repeatability of the test, a necessity for both clinical practice and research situations. A more reproducible technique of BUT measurement has been advocated: the instillation of a fixed amount of fluorescein (1 or 2 µl) of a 5 per cent sodium fluorescein solution by a laboratory pipette and the use of a barrier yellow filter (Schott-filter OG 530) with the biomicroscope to increase contrast. A Kodak Wratten 12 filter is also commonly used as well as interference filters (Cox and Fonn, 1991) for the same purpose.

Non-invasive break-up time measurement

Mengher *et al.* (1985a), following an original design by Lamble *et al.* (1976), developed a non-invasive technique for the assessment of precorneal tear film break-up time without the use of fluorescein (NIBUT). Their method is based on observing changes in the specular image of a grid pattern projected on to the open eye. A distortion of the grid line represents local thinning and discontinuity represents a break in the tear film. The time required for the appearance of the first discontinuity in the grid pattern is taken as a measure of tear film break-up.

Patel *et al.* (1985) observed the first catoptric image produced by a Bausch & Lomb keratometer (Figure 3.6) and measured the time taken for that image to become diffuse following the blink. They termed this measurement tear thinning time (TTT). TTT was also measured 3 minutes after fluorescein instillation, as well as BUT immediately after instillation.

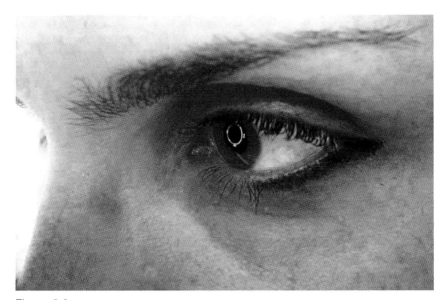

Figure 3.6

They found an average TTT of 18.0 ± 6.5 s and a reduction of 3.6 s due to the instillation of fluorescein. BUT showed greater values (22.7 ± 6.8 s), which may be due to the immediate effect of fluorescein on the tear film.

Mengher *et al.* (1985a) reported NIBUT in a normal population of 47.9 ± 5.3 s for the right eye (range 4–214 s) and 35.1 ± 3.2 s for the left eye (range 4–150 s). They found 62 per cent of observations to be >20 s in normal subjects compared to 37 per cent in dry eye patients, 33 per cent of whom exhibited a NIBUT <5 s. These authors also showed that fluorescein instillation significantly decreased tear film stability, as 64.7 per cent of NIBUT measured after instillation was <30 s compared to 80 per cent in the control eyes. Tear film stability recovered 10–20 minutes after fluorescein instillation (Mengher *et al.*, 1985b).

The HIR-CAL grid is a non-invasive test of tear film stability named after its inventors (Hirji *et al.*, 1989). It consists of a modified Bausch & Lomb keratometer where the mires have been replaced by a white grid on

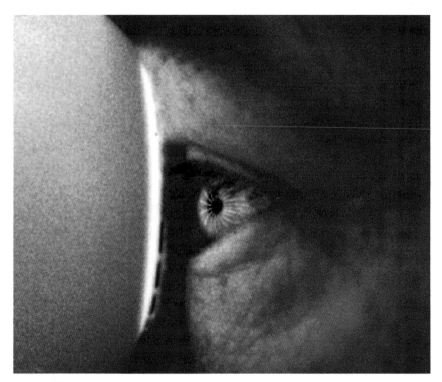

Figure 3.7

a black background. The image of the grid is reflected by the tear film and the appearance of distortion in the reflected pattern denotes a break. The time between a blink and a break is recorded as tear thinning time (TTT) and the mean of five measurements is calculated. The test has been used for research purposes but is not available commercially. When the standard keratometer mires on their own are observed they cover too small an area of the cornea to be an effective measure of tear film stability. The Loveridge Grid (Evans Instruments) is a hand-held instrument based on the Klein keratoscope where the concentric rings are replaced with an illuminated grid (Loveridge, 1995).

The Tearscope Plus allows the measurement of NIBUT by two techniques: a direct, non-invasive method by observing the break against the white background produced by the instrument; and indirectly by observing the deformation of rings or grid patterns inserted within the illuminated inner surface of the instrument (Figure 3.7).

Use of staining agents in clinical practice

A variety of stains have been employed in the study of the tear film and in routine ophthalmological, optometric and contact lens practice. A primary use has been in the detection of areas of epithelial compromise (punctate staining), and the presence of degenerated or dead cells. The BUT test makes use of stains to study the stability of the tear film. The most popular staining agents used routinely are sodium fluorescein and rose bengal. Lissamine green is a possible alternative to rose bengal.

Sodium fluorescein

Fluorescein sodium is a water-soluble dye of yellow-green coloration that can be excited by illumination with near ultraviolet light such as that produced by 'cobalt blue' filters. In practice, the blue filter of the biomicroscope and a yellow barrier filter are the most suitable combination. Maximum fluorescence is obtained for a concentration of $0.08\,g/\mu l$ and it is necessary to observe the staining after a few minutes for maximum effect. Several factors affect the fluorescence of fluorescein, in particular the concentration and the pH of the solution. Fluorescein accumulates in the intercellular spaces resulting from discontinuity in the corneal epithelium. The thickness of the tear film and its integrity can be assessed by the intensity of the coloration over the ocular surface. Patients with reduced tear volume and tear film thickness usually exhibit a less intense fluorescence despite repeated instillations. A normal tear film should exhibit an even and uniform green background. Thinning of the film becomes visible as a localized loss of fluorescence, which is usually followed by the appearance of a break. Epithelial fluorescein staining secondary to dry eye conditions and other ocular surface diseases is readily seen (Witcher, 1987). Apparently normal eyes can also exhibit staining (Korb and Korb, 1970; Norn, 1970). Sequential corneal staining has been advocated as a more sensitive technique for its predictive value of epithelial complication (Korb and Hermann, 1979). However, normal eyes can also exhibit staining when a sequential technique is used (Caffery and Josephson, 1991) and daily variations may occur (Josephson and Caffery, 1992).

Rose bengal

Rose bengal is a water-soluble dye which stains degenerated and dead cells and mucous fibrils (Norn, 1972). The stain produces a punctate coloration along the lacrimal rivus, known as the line of Marx, which is

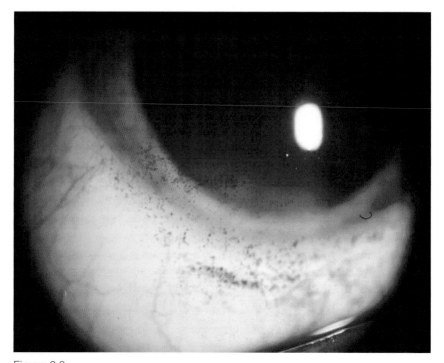

Figure 3.8

probably due to pronounced cell degeneration in this area. One per cent rose bengal is preferred as the irritation increases with higher concentrations. Its use as a diagnostic tool for dry eye is longstanding (Stenstam, 1947; Sjögren, 1950). Van Bijsterveld (1969) introduced numerical scoring for the intensity of rose bengal staining of the conjunctiva (both medial and lateral bulbar) and cornea.

In KCS, staining appears mostly in the area not covered by the eyelid (Figure 3.8). Most clinicians use a concentration of 1 per cent and instil one drop in the lower conjunctiva. Alternatively, strips impregnated with the stain can be wetted with saline and then applied, but it is not possible to control the concentration when this method is used. Because of the stinging that rose bengal produces, small amounts or greater dilution can be used for routine examination of prospective contact lens wearers.

In contact lens practice, the main use of rose bengal is to assess superficial damage during fitting or after prolonged wear. The uses of various other stains and combinations of stains have been well documented by Norn (1983) but have found little acceptance in routine ophthalmological, optometric or contact lens practice.

Recording of vital staining

Many classification systems exist to record staining since it appears in a variety of shapes, locations and intensities and can be categorized by appearance, type and severity. In the Van Bijsterveld scoring method (1969) the ocular surface is separated into three sections (cornea, medial and lateral bulbar conjunctiva), each of which is graded 1–3 according to severity. A score of 3.5 or higher indicates a pathological finding and differentiates between normal staining and the presence of KCS. This system remains the most widely used in ophthalmology.

Classification into seven types of abraded surfaces (arcuate abrasions, punctate, superficial, deep epithelial, linear, limbal, and superficial conjunctival); four types of staining (punctate, diffuse, line and dimple); and three levels of severity (superficial, moderate and deep).

It is also convenient to divide the cornea into areas. Begley *et al.* (1992) proposed five areas: central, superior, inferior, nasal and temporal. Four grades of punctate staining (<4 spots, 5–10 spots, 10–25 spots or >26 spots) have also been described (Begley *et al.*, 1992). The recording method used should help to differentiate between aetiologies such as drying, mechanical, toxic, allergic, physiological or infectious.

More recent grading systems in widespread use (CCLRU or Efron scales) utilize a combination of all of these recording techniques to improve their reliability and precision.

Measurement of tear secretion

Tear flow – the Schirmer test

Tear production rate, or tear flow, is of prime importance in maintaining a normal, wet eye. Marquardt (1982) found that tear film stability decreases with age in relation to the decrease in tear flow, although this finding is now in doubt. The tear flow rate was first measured and referred to as tear flow in 1903 by Schirmer when he used filter paper to collect the tear secretion of patients whose lacrimal sacs had been removed. Using this method, he collected 0.5–0.75 g over a 16-hour

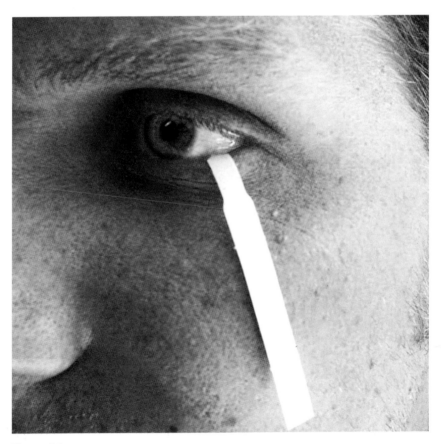

Figure 3.9

period, which corresponds roughly to 0.6–0.8 µl per minute. However, subsequent studies have produced widely differing results. These variations are mainly due to the experimental techniques for tear collection and the methods used to evaluate the results.

The Schirmer test uses a strip of filter paper 35 mm long and 5 mm wide which is bent at one end and placed in the lower conjunctival sac about one-third of the palpebral width from the temporal canthus (Figure 3.9). The strip is inserted in a dry state and induces some level of irritation and reflex tearing. It relies on the presence of a good tear meniscus to act as a reservoir from which fluid can be drawn and absorbed onto the paper. Conjunctival folds in this area may further influence the measurement. It is commonly accepted that < 5 mm of wetting in 5 minutes is a sign of a pathological dry eye, and 5–10 mm suggests a borderline dry eye, while > 10 mm represents a more normal state of lacrimal secretion.

Holly *et al.* (1986) demonstrated that the initial insertion of the strip induces a high rate of secretion which decreases in an exponential fashion towards a lower final rate. In dry eye subjects they found that the initial rate does not decrease significantly, but in KCS patients the final secretion rate is much lower and the secretion decay much faster. Reflex lacrimation may increase the tear volume by a factor of 100 (Maurice, 1980).

To date, five main techniques have been used to measure tear flow:

1. The Schirmer test, using collection by a filter paper or cotton thread
2. Dye dilution tests, using fluorescein
3. Tear flow calculation techniques
4. Slit-lamp fluorophotometry
5. Radioactive tracers.

While the Schirmer tear test is used clinically, the remaining four tests have been mainly used in research applications.

Phenol red thread test

Modifications to the Schirmer test can be made by replacing the filter strip with a fine cotton thread stained with phenol red. A change of coloration from orange to red revealed the length of the thread wetted by the alkali tears. The thread is inserted into the lower lacrimal lake for 15 s and a tear production deficiency is suspected when < 10 mm of thread is wetted. In view of its minimally invasive nature, the reflex lacrimation is reduced (Figure 3.10). A commercial version of the test has been available in Japan since the early 1980s and in the USA and has recently become available in the UK.

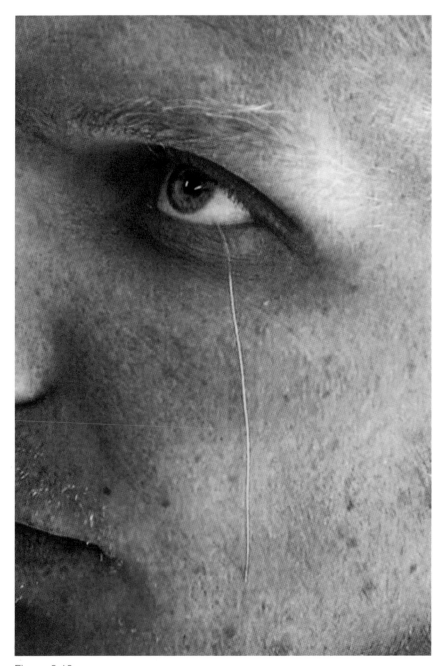

Figure 3.10

Tear dilution tests

In these tests the tear film is stained with rose bengal and fluorescein and examined after five minutes to detect the dilution of the dyes as disclosed by a change in colour of the meniscus. A red colour indicates a dry eye, yellow a normal eye, while a weak orange colour is the limit of normal dilution (Norn, 1965). Xu *et al.* (1995) introduced a Tear Function Index (TFI) which is calculated by dividing the Schirmer value in mm by the tear clearance rate (the dilution expressed as a fraction of the tear volume). Dry eye is indicated in TFI values < 96.

Protein assays

The lactoplate test uses a small filter paper disc placed in the lower cul-de-sac for several minutes to collect the patient's tear secretion (Figure 3.11). The disc is then transferred to a receptacle containing an immunoreactive gel where a precipitation ring is formed over a three-day period. The size of the ring is proportional to the lactoferrin concentration of the sample collected (Figure 3.12).

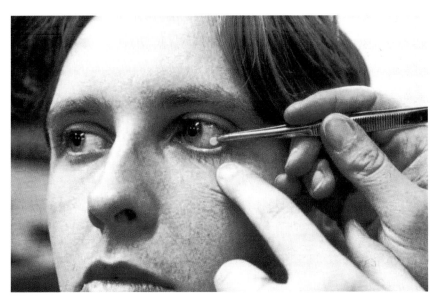

Figure 3.11

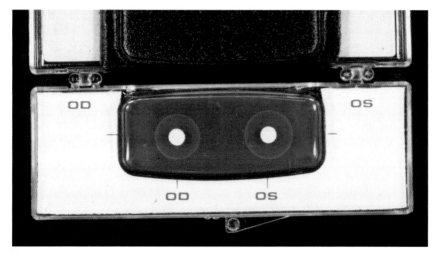

Figure 3.12

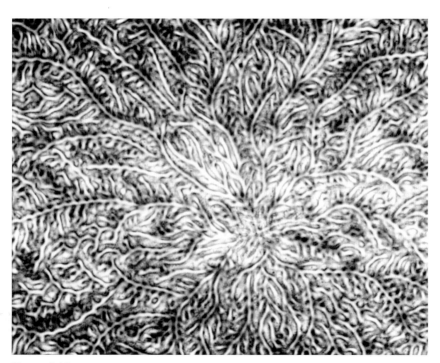

Figure 3.13

Tear ferning test

Tear film composition affects the way in which a collected sample dries on a glass slide. This test is based on mucus ferning patterns that have been used in cervical smear testing. Tears are collected with a glass capillary and placed on a glass slide and left to dry at room temperature. The sample is then observed in white light or by polarized microscopy and classified into four grades according to its appearance following crystallization. The tears of dry eye patients exhibit less ferning than those of normal patients (Figures 3.13, 3.14). Although the patterns produced are known as mucous ferning, the test may reflect the quality of tear protein profile. As a simple test complimentary to other techniques it may find acceptance in general optometric practice.

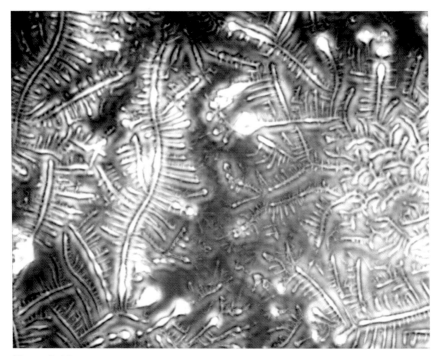

Figure 3.14

Conclusions

All the tests available for assessing the tear film and tear secretions must be used as part of a complete routine in order to determine with greater precision both the presence and severity of the dry eye. A suggested sequence of testing follows:

1. A comprehensive patient history and symptoms should be recorded, preferably using a written questionnaire
2. As the tear film is a very fragile structure, non-invasive tests should always be carried out first. Observation of the superficial lipid layer and NIBUT measurement can be used to initiate the examination
3. The lids may then be manipulated to determine if meibomian secretion can be digitally expressed
4. Slit-lamp observation of the lids and examination for conjunctival hyperaemia, preferably using appropriate grading scales, should follow
5. More invasive tests, such as Schirmer or cotton thread tests, can then be carried out, and tests of composition of the tear secretion or its kinetics used to refine the diagnosis
6. Tests using stains (fluorescein, rose bengal and lissamine green) for the ocular surface should be performed last in view of their effect on tearing and on the composition of the tear film.

In a busy practice, not all tests can be performed on all patients and it is the role of the practitioner to choose which tests to use routinely and which ones to have available for further investigation.

Acknowledgement

Illustrations in this chapter courtesy of Jennifer Craig.

References and further reading

Baum, J. L. (1973) Systemic diseases associated with tear deficiencies. *Int. Ophthalmol. Clin.*, **13,** 157–184.

Begley, C. G., Weirich, B., Benak, J. and Pence, N.A. (1992) Effect of rigid gas permeable contact lens solutions on the human corneal epithelium. *Optom. Vis Sci.*, **69,** 347.

Bron, A. J. (1985) Prospects for the dry eye. *Trans. Ophthalmol. Soc. UK*, **104**, 801–826.

Caffery, B. E. and Josephson, J. E. (1991) Corneal staining after sequential instillations of fluorescein over 30 days. *Optom. Vis. Sci.*, **68**, 467.

Clark, B. A. J. (1973) Some experiments in corneal interferometry. *Aust. J. Optom.*, **56**, 448–453.

Clark, B. A. J. and Carney, L. G. (1971) Refractive index and reflectance of the anterior surface of the cornea. *Am. J. Optom.*, **48**, 333–343.

Cox, I. and Fonn, D. (1991) Interference filters to eliminate the surface reflex and improve contrast during fluorescein photography. *Int. Cont. Lens Clin.*, **18 Sept**, 178–180.

Craig, J. P. and Tomlinson, A. (1997) Importance of the lipid layer in human tear film stability and evaporation. *Optom. Vis. Sci.*, **74**, 8–13.

Damato, B. E., Allan, D., Murray, S. B. and Lee, W. R. (1984) Senile atrophy of the human lacrimal gland: the contribution of chronic inflammatory disease. *Br. J Ophthalmol.*, **68**, 674–680.

Dilly, P. N. and Mackie, I. S. (1981) Surface changes in the anaesthetic conjunctiva in man with special reference to the production of mucus from non-goblet cell source. *Br. J. Ophthalmol.*, **65**, 833–842.

Doughty, M. J., Fonn, D., Richter, D. *et al.* (1997) A patient questionnaire approach to estimating the prevalence of dry eye symptoms in patients presenting to optometric practices across Canada. *Optom. Vis. Sci.*, **74(8)**, 624–631.

Ehlers, N. (1965) The pre corneal tear film. Biomicroscopical, histological and chemical investigations. *Acta Ophthalmol.*, **81(Suppl.)**, 5–136.

Fischer, F. P. (1928) Über die Darstellung der Hornhaut – Oberfläche und ihrer Veränderung im Reflexbild. *Arch. Augenheilk*, **98**, 1–84.

Forst, I. G. (1976) Experiments with the tear film BUT. *Optician*, **Jan(Suppl.)**.

Forst, I. G. (1978) Stabilitá della pellicola lacrimale e tollerabilitá di una lente a contacto. *L'ottico*, **178**, 16–25.

Fullard, R. D. and Snyder, C. (1995) Expanded Dry Eye Patient Questionnaire. In *Anterior Segment Complications of Contact Lens Wear* (ed. J. A. Silbert), New York, Churchill Livingstone, pp. 12–14.

Guillon, J.-P. (1982) Tear film photography and contact lens wear. *J. Br. Cont. Lens Assoc.*, **5(2)**, 84–87.

Guillon, J.-P. (1986) Tear film structure and contact lenses. In *The Preocular Tear Film in Health, Disease, and Contact Lens Wear* (ed. F. J. Holly), Lubbock, Dry Eye Institute, pp. 914–939.

Guillon, J.-P. (1990) Tear film structure of the contact lens wearer. PhD Thesis dissertation. The City University, London.

Guillon, J.-P. and Guillon, M. (1988a) Tear film examination of the contact lens patient. *Contax*, **May**, 14–18.

Guillon, J.-P. and Guillon, M. (1994) The role of tears in contact lens performance and its measurement. In *Contact Lens Practice* (eds M Guillon and M Ruben), London, Chapman and Hall, pp. 453–484.

Guillon, M. and Guillon, J.-P. (1988b) The status of the pre-soft lens tear film during overnight wear. *Am. J. Optom. Physiol. Opt.*, **65**, 40.

Guillon, M. and Guillon, J.-P. (1988c) Pre-lens tear film characteristics of high Dk rigid gas permeable lenses. *Am. J. Optom. Physiol. Opt.*, **65**, 73.

Guillon, M., Guillon, J.-P., Mapstone, V. and Dwyer, S. (1989) Rigid gas permeable lenses in vivo wettability. *Transactions of the British Contact Lens Association Conference*, London, Wolfe, 24–26.

Guillon, J.-P., Guillon, M. and Malgouyres, S. (1990) Desiccation staining with hydrogel lenses: tear film and contact lens factors. *Ophthalmol. Physiol. Opt.*, **10**, 343–350.

Guillon, M., Allary, J.-C., Guillon, J.-P. and Osborn, G. (1992) Clinical management of regular replacement. Part 1. Selection of replacement frequency. *ICLC*, **19**, 104–120.

Haberich, F. J. (1982) The stability of the precorneal tear film. In *15th Contact Lens Congress Aschaffenburg, March 1982*, Aschaffenburg, Titmus Eurocon Kontaktlinsen Gmbh & Co., pp. 17–45.

Hamano, H., Hamano, T., Hamano, T. *et al.* (1980a) Break-up of the pre-corneal tear film on a dendritic keratitis. *Fol. Ophthalmol. Japan*, **31**, 1071–1074.

Hamano, H., Hori, M., Kawabe, H. *et al.* (1980b): Clinical applications of biodifferential interference microscope. *Cont. Intraoc. Lens Med. J.*, **6(3)**, 229–235.

Hill, R. M. (1981) Laboratory studies. In *Complications of Contact Lenses* (ed. D. Miller and P. F. White), *Int. Ophthalmol. Clin.*, **21(2)**, 223–236.

Hirji, N., Patel, S. and Callender, M. (1989) Human tear film pre-rupture phase time (TP-RPT) – a non-invasive technique for evaluating the precorneal tear film using a novel keratometer mire. *Ophthal. Physiol. Opt.*, **9**, 139–142.

Hoh, H., Schirra, F., Kienecker, C. and Ruprecht, K. W. (1995) Lid-parallel conjunctival fold (LIPCOF) and dry eye: a diagnostic tool for the contactologist. *Contactologia*, **17E**, 104–117.

Holly, F. J. (1978) Surface chemical evaluation of artificial tears and their ingredients. I. Interfacial activity. *Cont. Intraoc. Lens Med. J.*, **4(2)**, 14–31.

Holly, F. J. (1980) Tear film physiology. *Am. J. Optom. Physiol. Opt.*, **57(4)**, 252–257.

Holly, F. J. (1981) Tear film physiology and contact lens wear. I. Pertinent aspects of tear film physiology. *Am. J. Optom. Physiol. Opt.*, **58(4)**, 324–330.

Holly, F. J. and Lemp, M. A. (1977) Tear physiology and dry eyes. *Surv. Ophthalmol.*, **22**, 69–87.

Holly, F. J., Beebe, W. E. and Esquivel, E. D. (1986) Lacrimation kinetics in human as determined by a novel technique. In *The Preocular Tear Film in Health, Disease, and Contact Lens Wear* (ed. F. J. Holly), Lubbock, Dry Eye Institute, pp. 76–88.

Josephson, J. E. (1983) Appearance of the pre ocular tear film lipid layer. *Am. J. Optom. Physiol. Opt.*, **60**, 883–887.

Josephson, J. E. and Caffery, B. E. (1992) Corneal staining characteristics after sequential instillations of fluorescein. *Optom. Vis. Sci.*, **69**, 570.

Kilp, H., Schmid, E. and Vogel, A. (1982) Tränenfilm Untersuchungen in Spiegelbezirk. *Klin. Mbl. Augenheilk.*, **180**, 49–52.

Klein, M. (1949) The lacrimal strip and the precorneal film in cases of Sjögren's syndrome. *Br. J. Ophthalmol.*, **33**, 387–388.

Knoll, H. and Walters, H. (1985) Pre-lens tear film specular microscopy. *Int. Cont. Lens Clin.*, **12(1)**, 30.

Korb, D. and Hermann, J. P. (1979) Corneal staining subsequent to sequential fluorescein instillations. *J. Am. Optom. Assoc.*, **50,** 316.

Korb, D. R. and Korb, J. M. E. (1970) Corneal staining prior to contact lens wearing. *J. Am. Optom. Assoc.*, **41(3)**, 228–232.

Korb, D. R., Greiner, J. and Glonek, T. (1997) Tear film lipid layer formation: implication for contact lens wear. *Optom. Vis. Sci.*, **73(3)**, 189–192.

Lamble, J. W., Gilbert, D. and Ashford, J. J. (1976) The break-up time of artificial preocular films on the rabbit cornea. *J. Pharm. Pharmacol.*, **28,** 450.

Lamberts, D. W., Foster, C. and Perry, H. P. (1979) Schirmer test after topical anaesthesia and the tear meniscus height in normal eyes. *Arch. Ophthalmol.*, **97(6)**, 1082–1085.

Lee, W. R., Murray, S. N., Williamson, S. and McKean, D. C. (1981) Human conjunctival surface mucins: a quantitative study of normal and diseased (KCS) tissues. *Graef. Arch. Ophthalmol.*, **245,** 209–221.

Lemp, M. A. (1995) Report of the National Eye Institute/industry workshop on clinical trials in dry eyes. *CLAO. J.*, **Oct. 21,** 221–232.

Lemp, M. A. and Hamill, J. R. (1973) Factors affecting tear film break-up in normal eyes. *Arch. Ophthalmol.*, **89(2)**, 103–105.

Lemp, M. A., Dohlman, C. H. and Holly, F. J. (1970) Corneal desiccation despite normal tear volume. *Ann. Ophthalmol.*, **2,** 258–261.

Loveridge, R. (1995) Breaking up is hard to do? *Optom. Today,* **Nov. 15,** 18–24.

Lydon, D. P. M. and Guillon, J.-P. (1984) The integrity of the pre-lens tear film. In *The Frontier of Optometry*, Transactions of the First International Congress of the British College of Optometrists, April 11–14, pp. 106–135.

Marquardt, R. (1982) Untersuchungen zur Tranenfilmstabilitas. In *Chronische Conjunctivitis Trockenes Auge*, Wien-New York, Springer-Verlag.

Maurice, D. M. (1973) The dynamics and drainage of tears. In *The Preocular Tear Film and Dry Eye Syndromes* (eds F. J. Holly and M. A. Lemp), *Int. Ophthalmol. Clin.* **13(1),** 103–116.

Maurice, D. M. (1980) Structures and fluids involved in the penetration of topically applied drugs. *Int. Ophthalmol. Clin.*, **20,** 7–20.

McCulley, J. P. and Sciallis, G. F. (1977) Meibomian keratoconjunctivitis. *Am. J. Ophthalmol.*, **84(6)**, 788–793.

McDonald, J. E. (1968) Surface phenomena of tear films. *Trans. Am. Ophthalmol. Soc.*, **66,** 905–939.

McDonald, J. E. (1969) Surface phenomena of the tear film. *Am. J. Ophthalmol.*, **67(1)**, 56–64.

McDonald, J. E. and Brubaker, S. (1971) Meniscus induced thinning of tear films. *Am. J. Ophthalmol.*, **72(1)**, 139–146.

McMonnies, C. W. (1986) Key questions in a dry eye history. *J. Am. Optom. Assoc.*, **57,** 512–517.

McMonnies, C. W. and Ho, A. (1986) Marginal dry eye diagnosis: history versus biomicroscopy. In *The Preocular Tear Film in Health, Disease and Contact Lens Wear* (ed. F. J. Holly), Lubbock, Dry Eye Institute, pp. 32–40.

McMonnies, C. W. and Ho, A. (1987a) Patient history in screening for dry eye conditions. *J. Am. Optom. Assoc.*, **58,** 296.

McMonnies, C. W. and Ho, A. (1987b) Responses to a dry eye questionnaire from a normal population. *J. Am. Optom. Assoc.*, **58,** 588.

Mengher, L. S., Bron, A. J., Tonge, S. R. and Gilbert, D. J. (1985a) A non-invasive instrument for the clinical assessment of the pre-corneal tear film stability. *Curr. Eye Res.*, **4**, 1–8.

Mengher, L. S., Bron, A. J., Tonge, S. R. and Gilbert, D. J. (1985b) Effect of fluorescein instillation on the pre-corneal tear film stability. *Curr. Eye Res.*, **4**, 9–11.

Norn, M. S. (1965) Tear secretion in normal eyes. *Acta Ophthalmol.*, **43(4)**, 567–573.

Norn, M. S. (1969) Desiccation of the pre corneal film. I. Corneal wetting time. *Acta Ophthalmol.*, **47(4)**, 865–880.

Norn, M. S. (1970) Micropunctate fluorescein vital staining of the cornea. *Acta Ophthalmol.*, **48**, 108.

Norn, M. S. (1972) Vital staining of the cornea and conjunctiva. *Acta Ophthalmol. (Kbh)*, **113(Suppl.)**, 9–66.

Norn, M. S. (1979) Semi-quantitative interference study of fatty layer of pre-corneal film. *Acta Ophthalmol. (Kbh)*, **57**, 766–774.

Norn, M. S. (1983) Studies of surface phenomena. In *External Eye: Methods of Examination*, 2nd edn, Copenhagen, Scriptor, pp. 80–92.

Norn, M. S. (1985) Meibomian orifices and Marx's line studied by triple vital staining. *Acta Ophthalmol.*, **63**, 698–700.

Olsen, T. (1985) Reflectometry of the precorneal film. *Acta Ophthalmol.*, **63**, 432–438.

Patel, S., Murray, D., McKenzie, A. *et al.* (1985) Effect of fluorescein on tear break-up time and on tear thinning time. *Am. J. Optom. Physiol. Opt.*, **62(3)**, 188–190.

Port, M. J. A. and Asaria, T. S. (1990) The assessment of human tear volume. *J. Br. Cont. Lens Assoc.*, **13(1)**, 76–82.

Rengstorff, R. H. (1974) The precorneal tear film: break-up time and location in normal subjects. *Am. J. Optom. Physiol. Opt.*, **51**, 765–769.

Robboy, M. and Osborn, G. (1988) The response of marginal dry eye lens wearers to a dry eye survey. *Cont. Lens J.*, **17(1)**, 8–9.

Rolando, M., Baldi, F. and Calabria, G. A. (1986) Tear mucous ferning test in keratoconjunctivitis sicca. In *The Preocular Tear Film in Health, Disease and Contact Lens Wear* (ed. F. J. Holly), Lubbock, Dry Eye Institute, pp. 203–210.

Rolando, M., Terragna, F., Giordano, G. and Calabria, G. (1990) Conjunctival surface damage distribution in keratoconjunctivitis sicca. An impression cytology study. *Ophthalmologica*, **200**, 170–176.

Rolando, M., Macri, A., Alongi, S. *et al.* (1997) Use of a questionnaire for the diagnosis of tear film related ocular surface disease. In *Lacrimal Gland, Tear Film and Dry Eye Syndromes* (ed. D. Sullivan), New York, Plenum Press (in press).

Schirmer, O. (1903) Studien zur Physiologie und Pathologie der Tränenabsonder-ung und Tränenabfuhr. *Graef. Arch. Ophthalmol.*, **56**, 197–291.

Schuller, W., Young, W. and Hill, R. M. (1972) Clinical measurements of the tears: viscosity. *Am. J. Optom. Assoc.*, **43**, 1358–1361.

Sjögren, H. (1950) Quelques problems concernant la keratoconjonctivite seche et le syndrome de KCS. *Ann. Ocul. Fr.*, **183**, 500–514.

Stenstam, T. (1947) On occurrence of keratoconjunctivitis sicca in cases of rheumatoid arthritis. *Acta. Med. Scand.*, **127**, 139–148.

Stodtmeister, R., Kessler, K. F. and Schlörer, J. (1983) Die Tränenfilmaufreißzeit bei Unterschiedlicher Anfärbung. *Klin. Mbl. Augenheilk.*, **183**, 110–114.

Taylor, H. R. (1980) Studies on tear film in climatic droplet keratopathy and pterygium. *Arch. Ophthalmol.*, **98**, 86–88.

Terry, J. E. (1984) Eye disease of the elderly. *J. Am. Optom. Assoc.*, **55**, 23–29.

Vanley, G. T., Leopold, I. H. and Gregg, T. H. (1977) Interpretation of tear film break-up time. *Arch. Ophthalmol.*, **95**, 445–448.

Van Bijsterveld, O. P. (1969) Diagnostic tests in the sicca syndrome. *Arch. Ophthalmol.*, **82**, 10–14.

Witcher, J. P. (1987) Clinical diagnosis of the dry eye. *Int. Ophthalmol. Clin.*, **27**, 7.

Wolff, E. (1946) The muco-cutaneous junction of the lid margin and the distribution of the tear fluid. *Trans. Ophthalmol. Soc. UK*, **66**, 291–308.

Wright, P. (1971) Diagnosis and management of dry eyes. *Trans. Ophthalmol. Soc. UK*, **91**, 119–128.

Xu, K., Yagi, Y., Toda, I. and Tsubota, K. (1995) Tear Function Index: a new measure of dry eye. *Arch. Ophthalmol.*, **113**, 84–88.

4 Time and the tear film

Alan Tomlinson and Jennifer Craig

Introduction

Ageing is a normal biological process and occurs on a cellular and tissue level throughout life (Unger, 1967). Gerontology and geriatrics are concerned with the period when the deleterious effects of ageing manifest themselves in the decline of functional capacity and an increase in mortality rate. The decline in functions of the body differ; for example, ageing may be demonstrated to begin in the third decade of life (Strehler, 1962) for the visual and auditory systems and for some

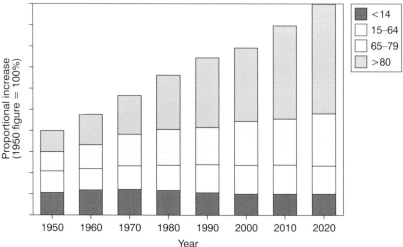

Figure 4.1 Proportional change in various age groups in the European population in the time period 1950–2020 (modified from data in deJong-Gierveld and Solinge H (eds), 1995, Populations Studies 29, Council of Europe Press

muscle activity, endocrine function and connective tissue elasticity. Geriatrics is principally concerned with the accumulated ageing processes at later stages of life – those generally described as senescence. Senescence and ageing involve two modalities, genetic constitution and environmental influences, although the effects of these are virtually impossible to separate.

Most ageing processes lead to a loss in function but the ultimate end result of ageing is death. Every death is a result of accident; death due to senile changes is extremely rare. In old age the lethal threshold falls until, in theory, the most trivial accident or disease can be a cause of death (Unger, 1967). As the population ages this means increasing numbers of people reach an age which approaches the biblical lifespan for mankind. In view of the anticipated demographic bulge in the older population in the second decade of this century (Figure 4.1), governments have put considerable funds into research on ageing in an attempt to increase lifespan and maintain quality of life.

Dry eye (keratoconjunctivis sicca)

The ageing process may affect the tear film. Dry eye or keratoconjunctivitis sicca (KCS), although not a fatal condition, is one which may be a result of the normal changes in the biological processes which occur with time and is the commonest cause of aqueous-deficient non-Sjögren's dry eye (NSDE). This condition is caused by a gradual infiltration of the lacrimal gland with lymphocytes that destroy the acinar and ductal tissue (Stasior and Roen, 1994). The next most common cause of dry eye is Sjögren's syndrome (SSDE), in which there is autoimmune disease leading to destruction of the lacrimal gland and impairment of reflex tear secretion (Bron et al., 1997).

There is a general presumption that pathological dry eye (KCS) is an age-related condition (Ungar, 1967; Lawrence, 1970; Medsger and Masi, 1985; Bron et al., 1997), but the literature is somewhat ambivalent. Defining the condition is difficult and depends on the diagnostic criteria applied and the composition of the study population. Definition by symptomatology alone may not be sufficient. A recent survey of the prevalence of dry-eye symptoms among patients attending optometric practices across Canada (Doughty et al., 1997) found a bimodal distribution of 'dry eye' symptoms, with the highest proportion of symptoms reported in the 21–30 year age group. A decline in symptoms in the age groups from 40–70 years was found, with a rise again for age ranges above 70 years. A greater predominance of symptoms was found in females than in males.

Most of the recent studies have chosen to look at the frequency of KCS, and particularly Sjögren's syndrome, in elderly populations. Strickland *et al.* (1987) found in a population of older females (aged 63–92) that 39 per cent had symptoms and 24 per cent had abnormal Schirmer tear test results; 2 per cent were classified as having Sjögren's syndrome and 12 per cent as suspect. These latter figures compare with KCS estimates for the general population of between 0.05 and 0.2 per cent (Shearn, 1971). An autopsy study of 900 sequential individuals based on salivary gland biopsies reported a figure of 0.44 per cent (Shearn, 1971). Drosos *et al.* (1988) examined 62 elderly, apparently healthy volunteers, for evidence of primary Sjögren's syndrome and found three cases defined by lip biopsy scores greater than 2+ and other objective criteria. This gave a prevalence in his elderly population of 4.8 per cent.

In a study of 2500 subjects aged over 65 years, Schein *et al.* (1996) confirmed that the prevalence of dry eye was dependent on the criteria for diagnosis. Based on dry eye symptoms and a rose bengal score ≥ 5, a prevalence of 2 per cent was found; symptoms and a Schirmer test result ≤ 5 gave a prevalence of 2.2 per cent; and symptoms with rose bengal ≤ 5 or Schirmer ≤ 5 gave a prevalence of 3.5 per cent. For none of the groups, defined by these criteria, was age, gender or race a determining factor.

In a study of younger individuals (aged 30–60 years) in Scandinavia (Bjerrum, 1997), symptoms of dry eye and oral dryness were found to be very common. KCS was more frequent in persons aged 50–59 and was equally common in men or women. The frequency of KCS in persons aged 30–60 was dependent on the criteria applied. It was found to be 11 per cent according to the Copenhagen criteria (Manthorpe *et al.*, 1986) and 8 per cent according to the preliminary European criteria (Vitali *et al.*, 1993). The frequency of primary Sjögren's syndrome in persons aged 30–60 was shown to be between 0.2 per cent and 0.8 per cent according to the Copenhagen criteria (Manthorpe *et al.*, 1986), and between 0.6 per cent and 2.1 per cent according to the European criteria (Vitali *et al.*, 1993). The symptoms of dry eye were not found to increase significantly with age or gender. Bjerrum (1997) found that symptoms of dry eye were extremely frequent and in most cases could not be explained by the presence of KCS. But complaints of 'burning eyes' and 'sensations of oral dryness' were significantly correlated to the presence of KCS, making these the best predictors.

Most studies of the prevalence of primary Sjögren's syndrome have dealt with populations over 60 (Strickland *et al.*, 1987; Drosos *et al.*, 1988) but the study by Bjerrum (1997) attempted to define whether the condition existed earlier in life and remained undiagnosed for a number of years. They found only a few patients with early stages of the disease. Jacobsson *et al.* (1989) had found a 2.7 per cent incidence in persons aged

52–72 years. This compared with the 2 per cent found by Strickland (1987) in patients 63–99 years and led to the impression that although primary Sjögren's may be difficult to diagnose in the early stages, it is primarily a problem of older age, with frequency and severity increasing after the age of 50 years.

The inevitability of dry eye with ageing

This review of the ageing tear film will consider whether the progression towards the pathological dry eye is inevitable with age or if it is due to the intervention of a disease process. With advancing years, tear physiology is affected by genetic and environmental influences. Genetic predisposition to certain forms of disease, particularly systemic disease associated with ocular manifestations of dry eye, will be a factor in the development of the condition; however, there are also environmental factors in the modern world which are significant. Environmental pollutants, contact lens wear and medication which affects tear function can all lead to a predisposition to dry eye. To establish whether the development of dry eye is inevitable if a person lives long enough, it is useful to determine the age changes that take place in the tear physiology of persons defined as normal.

'Normal' age changes in tear physiology

A large number of studies have been carried out to determine the changes in tear composition that take place in individuals as they grow older (Table 4.1). These studies have concentrated mainly on the effect of age on the biophysical characteristics of the tear film and its chemistry. The results are ambivalent with respect to defining the normal effect of ageing on tears.

Tear production

The area in which there is the greatest consensus about the effects of age on tear physiology is that of reflex tear production. The Schirmer test has been used to measure this reflex tears in study samples with a range of ages. Decreased reflex tear production with age has been described (Henderson and Prough, 1950; Norn, 1965; McGill et al., 1984), particularly after the age of 40 years (Figure 4.2, Table 4.2). Mathers et al. (1996a) showed a similar change with automated, scanning fluorophotometry.

Table 4.1 Age changes in tear composition and biophysics

Study	N	Age range	Percentage female	Parameter	Technique	Age correlation Y/N
Henderson and Prough, 1950	231	16–67	51	Reflex tears	Schirmer test	Y
Norn, 1965	93 normals	<10–90	50	Tear secretion	Lac streak dilution test	Y, stable after 30 years old
Mishima et al., 1966	40	20–80		Tear flow	Fluorophotometry	Y
				Tear volume		N
Pietsch et al., 1973	460	10–60		Lysozyme	Plating	Y
Norn, 1974				BUT		N
Sen et al., 1976	50 normals	14–50	26	IgA	Radial immunoassay	N
Dohlman et al., 1976	39 normals, 31 dry eye	18–62		Protein, mucus, flow rate	Lowry technique, PAS stain, Pipette	N
Millodot, 1977	205 normals	7–80		Corneal sensitivity	Anaesthesiometer	Y; constant until 40 years
Furukawa and Polse, 1978	68 normals	15–63		Tear flow – reflex (?)	Fluorometry	Y
Avisar et al., 1979	143 normals	1–80		Lysozyme	Plating	N
Lamberts et al., 1979	265	12–80	46	Basal tear flow	Schirmer with anaesthesia	N

Table 4.1 continued

Study	N	Age range	Percentage female	Parameter	Technique	Age correlation Y/N
Marquandt et al., 1980				BUT		N
Sen et al., 1980	114	<15->60	51	Lysozyme	Immunodiffusion	N
Rolando et al., 1983	52 normals, 52 dry eye	28–71	35	Evaporation	Humidity detector	N
Mackie et al., 1984	54 normals	20–80		Lysozyme, lactoferrin; IgA, IgG, cerulosplasmin	ELISA	Y Lactoferrin, lysozyme; N IgA, IgG, ceruloplasmin
Seal et al., 1986	66 normals	20–80		Lysozyme, lactoferrin; IgA, IgG, ceruloplasmin	ELISA	Y Lactoferrin, lysozyme; N IgA, IgG, ceruloplasmin
McGill et al., 1984	55 normals	20–82		Tear protein components; Lysozyme, lactoferrin, IgG ceruloplasmin, IgA	ELISA	Y, lysozyme, lactoferrin, after 40 years; N, IgG, IgA, ceruloplasmin (Y, after age 40)
Patel et al., 1988	123 normals	8–80		Tear flow; Tear thinning time	Schirmer; Keratometer	Y
Andres et al., 1987	200 normals	11–72	72	BUT	Slit lamp	Slight change of 2 s in 15–60 years
Hamano et al., 1990	11 336 normals	<10–69		Tear volume	Phenol thread test	N for = 9 mm, Y for = 15 mm

Port et al., 1990	100 normals	16–25, 46–55	48	Tear meniscus height	Slit lamp	N
Kuppens, 1992	133 normals and glaucoma	30–70		TTR	Fluorophotometry	N
Tomlinson et al., 1994	47 normals	7–92	55	Evaporation	Relative temperature and humidity detector	N
Craig and Tomlinson, 1995	100 normals	17–75	50	Osmolality	Freezing point depression, osmometry	N, Y for females
Nelson, 1995–1996	Normals and DE	17–75	50	TTR	Fluorophotometry	
Mathers et al., 1996	72 normals	10–70+	70	Reflex flow	Schirmer	Y
				TTR	Fluorophotometry	N
				Tear volume	Fluorophotometry	Y
				MGF	Transillumination	Y
				Lipid volume	Expression	N
				Viscosity	Digital compression	Y
				Evaporation	Humidity detector	Y
				Osmolality	Freezing point depression	Y
					Osmometry	
Craig and Tomlinson, 1998	145 normals	13–75	45	Evaporation	Relative temperature and humidity	N, Y for osmolality in females
				BUT	Hircal grid	
				Reflex and basal tears	Gamma scintigraphy	

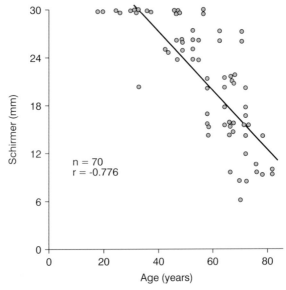

Figure 4.2 Relationship between modified Schirmer test results and age (McGill et al., 1984)

Table 4.2 Tear meniscus heights for young and older subjects (modified from data of Port and Asaria, 1990)

TMH results from 66 young subjects			TMH values for presbyopic group		
Mean of right and left eye (mm)			Mean of right and left eye (mm)		
	Primary	Up		Primary	Up
Mean	0.18	0.25	Mean	0.19	0.27
Median	0.18	0.25	Median	0.21	0.26
SD	0.03	0.05	SD	0.04	0.04
Minimum	0.11	0.15	Minimum	0.10	0.20
Maximum	0.26	0.40	Maximum	0.26	0.33

A reduction in reflex tear production may be attributable to the decreased corneal sensitivity observed with age (Millodot, 1977). Conversely, studies with a gamma scintigraphy device (Craig, 1995) and using a pipette technique (Dohlmann et al., 1976) did not show a similar decrease in reflex tearing during the initial phase of measurement.

Basal tear production has been investigated by a number of workers to determine its relationship to age. Lamberts et al. (1979) used the Schirmer

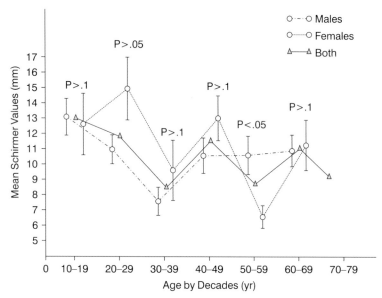

Figure 4.3 Schirmer test mean values according to decade, with anaesthesia (Lamberts *et al.*, 1979)

test with anaesthetic to determine basal flow rates and found they were unaffected by age (Figure 4.3). Tear turnover rates under basal conditions, measured by modern fluorophotometric techniques, confirm this absence of an age relationship (Kuppens *et al.*, 1992; Nelson, 1995; Mathers *et al.*, 1996a). A similar result is found when measurements of basal rates are taken by gamma scintigraphy (Craig, 1995). However, earlier measurements by modified slit-lamp fluorophotometry showed decreased tear flow rates with age (Mishima *et al.*, 1966; Furukawa and Polse, 1978). It is possible that these earlier techniques measured a combination of reflex and basal tear secretion.

Tear film stability

Tear film stability has been assessed by a number of invasive and non-invasive techniques for measuring tear break-up times. Andres *et al.* (1987) instilled fluorescein to measure tear film break-up and, with Patel and Farrell (1988), using a non-invasive technique, found a decrease in tear stability with age. However, this finding was not confirmed by the work of Norn (1974), Marquardt and Wenz (1980) or Craig and Tomlinson (1995, 1998) (Figure 4.4), all of whom found no decrease in stability with age using non-invasive assessment.

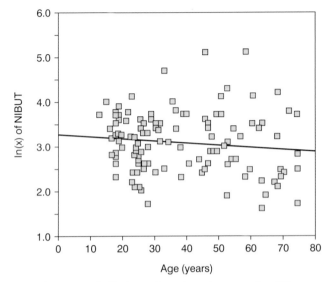

Figure 4.4 Transformed NIBUT data plotted against age for 125 normal subjects. No relationship was found (Craig, 1995)

Tear volume

Tear volume has been estimated by a number of techniques and the relation to age is again ambivalent. Mishima *et al.* (1966), using early fluorophotometric techniques, found no decrease in tear volume with age although Mathers *et al.* (1996a), with later techniques, did find a decrease with age. Port and Asaria (1990) found no decrease in tear volume as measured by inferior tear prism height (Table 4.2). Hamano *et al.* (1990), using the phenol red thread test, found no decrease with age for individuals with wetting lengths of ≤9 mm, but did find a decrease with age among those with wetting lengths > 15 mm.

Tear film evaporation

Tear film evaporation is a feature that is generally considered to be constant with age (Rolando and Refojo, 1983; Tomlinson and Giesbrecht, 1993; Craig, 1995), although Mathers *et al.* (1996a) found an increase in older individuals (Figure 4.5).

Tear osmolality

The osmolality of the tear film has been found to be constant throughout life by Craig and Tomlinson (1998) (Figure 4.6), but is reported as increasing with age by Mathers (1996a).

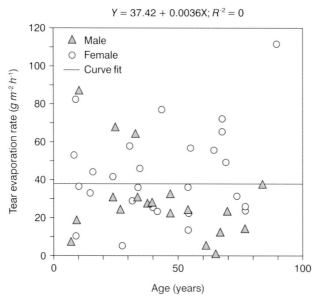

Figure 4.5 Tear evaporation rate with age. No significant correlation was found (Tomlinson *et al.*, 1993)

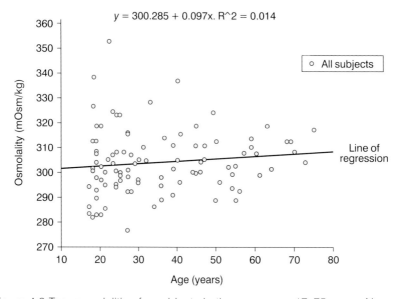

Figure 4.6 Tear osmolalities for subjects in the age range 17–75 years. No significant correlation was found with age when all male and female subjects were considered (Craig and Tomlinson, 1995)

Lipid layer characteristics

Mathers *et al.* (1996a) reported that tear film viscosity and lipid volume decreased with age, whereas Craig (1995) did not find a difference in the lipid layer structure or characteristics with age when assessed by interference fringe biomicroscopy.

A current view of the biophysics of the ageing tears

The ambivalent nature of the evidence presented by these various studies of tear biophysics in normal ageing populations may arise from several factors. The definition of 'normality' is not always clear. Most investigators use questionnaire assessment to determine study inclusion, but this may not be sufficiently rigorous (Bjerrum, 1997; Doughty *et al.*, 1997). Also, techniques of measurement vary, even when supposedly measuring the same feature. This is inevitable with the developments in technology over the 50 years covered by this review; however, it makes the comparison of results difficult.

Sample size and composition is also a major factor in accounting for the disparity in results. The difficulty of obtaining sufficiently large samples of individuals, particularly in the youngest and oldest age groups, makes the age ranges limited in many studies. Of the 27 studies listed in Table 4.2 only two have subjects older than 80, most limit their age range to the mid-70s and below 80 years (17) and six have distributions restricted to below 70 years. This means that estimates of true population trends from these samples are questionable. The gender bias inherent in some samples (Table 4.1) is another factor which may be significant in view of the importance of hormonal influences (Sullivan *et al.*, 1998a, 1998b) on tear physiology and in the aetiology of dry eye.

A relationship may be expected between tear production, stability, volume, evaporation, osmolality and lipid layer characteristics (Figure 4.7). Increased tear instability caused by an inadequate lipid layer (Craig and Tomlinson, 1997) will lead to increased tear evaporation and a decrease in tear volume in the eye. Tear volume will also fall in the event of decreased production. All of these factors will lead to increased tear osmolality. Crucial to this scenario for the ageing tear film is the rise in tear osmolality with age, since osmolality is the end product of changes in other tear characteristics. In view of the conflicting evidence, it is difficult to draw final conclusions on the 'natural' process of tear film ageing for the population as a whole. However, interim judgements can be made on the basis of current evidence.

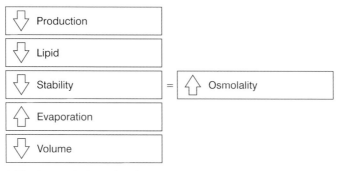

Figure 4.7 The inter-relationship of tear biophysical characteristics

From the literature, the majority view is that reflex tear production decreases with age but basal tear secretion rates are constant. Tear evaporation rate is also constant with age, as is tear volume, probably due to unchanging tear stability. If basal tear secretion, volume and evaporation rate do not decrease, then tear osmolality should remain constant as individuals age.

The major study which disagrees with this view of the normal, ageing tear film is that of Mathers *et al.* (1996a) who found decreased tear volume, increased evaporation and osmolality with age. An explanation for this may lie in the choice of sample in this study; of the 72 subjects tested, 51 (70 per cent) were female. Craig and Tomlinson (1995) found no increase in tear osmolality overall when a gender-balanced sample was considered. However, when females were considered independently of males, osmolality was found to increase with age. It should be noted that the values for 'older' females were within the range of normal and did not differ significantly from age-matched males, whereas young females had values well below the population average. The decreased osmolality in young females may be related to the increased rate of reflex tear production found for this group (Henderson and Prough, 1950). A recalculation of the Craig and Tomlinson (1995) data with a similar gender bias to that in the Mathers study reveals a significant relationship between osmolality and age (Figure 4.8) for all subjects ($r_2 = 0.163$, F = 18.31, $P = 0.0001$). This is due to the strong correlation of osmolality and age in females ($r_2 = 0.204$, F = 16.70, $P = 0.0001$), the males not showing any age relationship ($r_2 = 0.065$, F = 1.88, $P = 0.18$).

Tear composition

Evidence for the effect of age on tear composition is also ambivalent. Many find a decrease in tear lysozyme with age (Pietsch *et al.*, 1973; Mackie and

$$y = 299.95 + 0.11571x \quad R^{\wedge}2 = 0.065 \text{ (males)}$$
$$y = 291.46 + 0.23x \quad R^{\wedge}2 = 0.204 \text{ (females)}$$

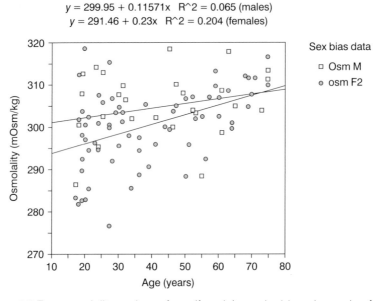

Figure 4.8 Tear osmolality and age for a (female) gender-biased sample of subjects aged from 17–75 years. A significant correlation for all subjects is shown in this biased sample. (Figure is derived from a recalculation of data previously reported in Craig and Tomlinson, 1995)

Seal, 1984; McGill *et al.*, 1984; Seal *et al.*, 1986), but this is an observation not confirmed by all (Dohlmann *et al.*, 1976; Avisar *et al.*, 1979; Sen and Sarin, 1980). A decrease in production of the other major lacrimal gland protein, lactoferrin, was also found by McGill *et al.* (1984) and Mackie and Seal (1984). A decrease in major lacrimal gland proteins with age would be consistent with decreased reflex lacrimation (Figure 4.9). The immunoglobulins IgG and IgA were found to remain constant (Sen *et al.*, 1976; Mackie and Seal, 1984; McGill *et al.*, 1984; Seal *et al.*, 1986) until later life when they apparently increase, probably due to an increased concentration with advancing age (McGill *et al.*, 1984). Caeruloplasmin showed a similar pattern of constancy followed by increasing concentration (Mackie and Seal, 1984; McGill *et al.*, 1984; Seal *et al.*, 1986).

Status of the 'old' tear film

Anecdoctal reports suggest that the incidence of dry eye increases with age (Norn, 1965; Bron *et al.*, 1997) although the vast majority of older persons do not have dry eye. The incidence of confirmed KCS (by

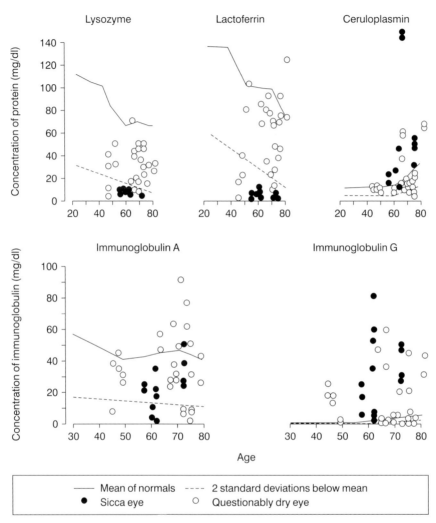

Figure 4.9 Tear protein levels in keratoconjunctivitis sicca and questionable dry eyes (Seal *et al.*, 1986)

objective clinical testing) varies from 0.05 per cent (Shearn, 1971) to 4.8 per cent (Drosos *et al.*, 1988). If symptoms alone are taken as an indicator of borderline and pathological dry eye, the incidence is much higher, rising to 40 per cent in some groups (includes those with lower ages) (Doughty *et al.*, 1997). In view of the other factors which might lead to symptoms of (borderline) dry eye, classification on the basis of sympto-matology alone is probably unreliable and a more rigorous clinical definition must be applied. The absence of dry eye pathology in most older individuals suggests that tear physiology may generally be adequate in later life. While it is probable that lacrimal gland function decreases with age, as evidenced by the reduction in reflex tear production and changes in tear composition, the tear film as a whole still appears to be functional. This may be explained by the majority view that the essential biophysical features of tear physiology, basal secretion, stability, volume, evaporation, lipid layer structure and osmolality, all remain fairly constant over time. Alternatively, these features may decline at a rate that it is insufficient to compromise function.

Another, potentially compensatory, mechanism for preserving functional tear performance in the older individual may be provided by changes in the rate of tear elimination from the eye with increasing age (Tomlinson and Giesbrecht, 1993). Reduced drainage from the eye would help to retain the fluid present. Dalgleish (1964) observed that the onset of idiopathic obstruction to lacrimal drainage occurs after the age of 35 and is more likely with age. Others have found an association between tear secretion and outflow in the eye (Norn, 1966; Kuppens et al., 1992). It has been shown that in the congenital absence of lid puncta there is almost a complete absence of lacrimation (Allen, 1968). These findings suggest the possibility of an autoregulation mechanism linking the production and drainage of lacrimal fluid (Francois et al., 1973). Recent experiments among a normal population undergoing punctal inclusion provides evidence of subsequent reductions in tear production (Tomlinson et al., 1998) (Figure 4.10).

A further factor which must be considered is the redundancy in the lacrimal system, which gives it great robustness in adverse conditions or situations of reduced capacity. Reflex tear flow occurs normally at just over $1\,\mu l/min$ (Norn, 1965) and can increase in response to stimuli by a factor of 100 times. An increase to a flow rate of $100\,\mu l/min$ can be contained within the eye without overflow if the increase in flow is gradual (Gasset et al., 1966). This indicates that the redundant drainage capacity of the system is 100 times greater than that required under normal conditions, a value confirmed by Maurice (1973). Reflex tear flow declines with age but this can reduce by a factor of four without discomfort (Stiewe, 1962; Wright and Mager, 1962). The normal tear volume in the eye is $7\,\mu l$, and rapid increases in volume up to $28\,\mu l$ can be accepted before epiphora occurs (Records, 1979). The buffering capacity of the tears is very good, with pH values of 7.1–8.6 being accepted without symptoms of discomfort (Records, 1979). The lipid film on the anterior surface of the tears remains intact with age, despite major changes in the glands responsible for its production. With increasing age the number of actively secreting meibomian glands decreases, so that by 80 years only half of the glands are active (Norn, 1987). In addition, only 45 per cent of all glands are active at one time, regardless of age

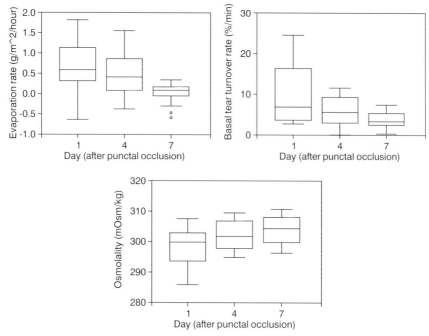

Figure 4.10 The effect of punctal occlusion on tear evaporation, turnover rate and osmolality. The data incorporated in these figures has been previously reported (Craig *et al.*, 1998)

(Norn, 1985). Tear stability as measured by tear break-up time is often in excess of 15 s (Andres *et al.*, 1987), much greater than the normal interblink period of 5 s. It is perhaps because of these inherent excess capacities of tear physiology that changes can occur with age without significantly compromising function.

Mathers *et al.* (1996b) developed a theoretical model for tear film function relating the biophysical characteristics of tears and lid features. This model is based on data from normal and dry eye populations and those with meibomian gland dysfunction. It depicts osmolality as the end result of other tear factors. For all subjects tear flow, evaporation and lipid function contribute significantly to this end result. In meibomian gland dysfunction, the contribution of tear flow to evaporation was enhanced. Mather's model is not markedly altered when the relationship of age to tear characteristics (Mathers *et al*, 1996b) is factored out. This suggests that the essential model describing the links between aspects of tear physiology is age-independent, so that a different model is not required for the older individual.

Tears in the ageing process

The decline in lacrimal gland function with age, caused by changes at the cellular level affecting secretion, may be placed in the context of the body's normal ageing process. Although it makes the lacrimal system more vulnerable, this change is not enough in itself to compromise tear physiology and result in pathological dry eye in the majority of older individuals. The maintenance of basal tear secretion rates, the relative robustness of tear film stability and the constancy of tear evaporation as a result of adequate (Norn, 1979), though reduced, lipid production (Norn, 1987; Hom *et al.*, 1990) allows most older persons to remain free of dry eye throughout life. When it occurs, pathological dry eye appears to be the direct result of the intervention of an additional factor: a disease process. This may be a process affecting the lacrimal system and tear production or the composition of the tears, resulting in instability and increased evaporation (Cohen *et al.*, 1997). It is often secondary to a systemic condition such as osteo- or rheumatoid arthritis, or Sjögren's syndrome. Predisposition to such conditions may be determined genetically as well as by exposure to environmental factors. Borderline dry eye, which accounts for symptoms and minor pathology in some cases of young and old patients, results directly from environmental factors of modern life, specifically the effect of modern drug therapies (Polak, 1987), industrial pollutants and contact lens wear (Tomlinson, 1992).

References

Allen, J. (1968) Congenital absence of the lacrimal punctum. *J. Pediatr. Ophthalmol.*, **5**, 176–178.

Andres, S. *et al.* (1987) Factors in pre-corneal tear film break-up time (TBUT) of contact lenses. *Int. Cont. Lens Clin.*, **14**, 103–107.

Avisar, R. *et al.* (1979) Lysosyme content of tears in patients with Sjögren's syndrome and rheumatoid arthritis. *Med. J. Ophthalmol.*, **87**, 148–151.

Bjerrum, K. B. (1997). Keratoconjunctivitis sicca in primary Sjögren syndrome in a Danish population aged 30–60 years. *Acta Ophthalmol.*, **75**, 281–286.

Bron, A. *et al.* (1997) The management of dry eyes. *Optician*, **214**, 13–25.

Cohen, E. S. *et al.* (1997) Punctal occlusion for dry eye. *Ophthalmology*, **104**, 1521–1524.

Craig, J. P. (1995) Tear physiology in the normal and dry eye. PhD Thesis, Glasgow Caledonian University.

Craig, J. P. and Tomlinson, A. (1995) Effect of age on tear osmolality. *Optom Vis, Sci.*, **72**, 713–717.

Craig, J. P. and Tomlinson, A. (1997) Importance of the lipid layer in human tear film stability and evaporation. *Optom. Vis. Sci.*, **74**, 8–13.

Craig, J. P. and Tomlinson, A. (1998) Age and gender effects on the normal tear film. In *Lacrimal Gland, Tear Film and Dry Eye Syndromes 2* (eds D. A. Sullivan, D. A. Dartt and M. A. Meneray). *Adv. Exp. Med. Biol.*, **438**, 411–415.

Dalgleish, R. (1964) Incidence of idiopathic acquired obstructions in the lacrimal drainage apparatus. *Br. J. Ophthalmol.*, **48**, 373–376.

Dohlmann, C. H. *et al.* (1976) The glycoprotein (mucus) content from normal and dry eye patents. *Exp. Eye Res.*, **22**, 359–365.

Doughty, M. J. *et al.* (1997) A patient questionnaire approach to estimating the prevalence of dry eye symptoms in patients presenting to optometric practices across Canada. *Optom. Vis. Sci.*, **74**, 624–631.

Drosos, A. A. *et al.* (1988) Prevalence of primary Sjögren's syndrome in an elderly population. *Br. J. Rheumatol.*, **27**, 123–127.

Francois, J. and Neetens, A. (1973) Tear flow in Man. *Am. J. Ophthalmol.*, **76**, 351–358.

Furukawa, R. and Polse, K. (1978) Changes in tear flow accompanying ageing. *Am. J. Optom. Vis. Optics*, **55**, 69–74.

Gassett, A. *et al.* (1966) Determination of tear flow and tear volume. *Invest. Ophthalmol.*, **5**, 264–276.

Hamano, T. *et al.* (1990) Tear volume in relation to contact lens wear and age. *CLAO J.*, **16**, 57–61.

Henderson, J. W. and Prough, W. A. (1950) Influence of age and sex on the flow of tears. *Arch. Ophthalmol.*, **43**, 224–228.

Hom, M. M. *et al.* (1990) Prevalence of meibomian gland dysfunction. *Optom. Vis. Sci.*, **67**, 710–712.

Jacobsson, L. T. H. *et al.* (1989) Dry eyes and dry mouth: an epidemiological study in Swedish adults with special reference to primary Sjögren syndrome. *J. Autoimmun.*, **2**, 521–527.

Kuppens, E. *et al.* (1992) Basal tear turnover and topical timolol in glaucoma patients and healthy controls. *Invest. Ophthalmol. Vis. Sci.*, **33**, 3442–3448.

Lamberts, D. *et al.* (1979) Schirmer's test after topical anaesthesia and the tear meniscus height in normal eyes. *Arch. Ophthalmol.*, **97**, 1082–1085.

Lawrence, J. S. (1970) The epidemiology of rheumatic diseases. In *Textbook of Rheumatic Diseases* (ed. W. S. C. Copeman), Edinburgh, E. S. Livingston, pp. 163–181.

Mackie, I. A. and Seal, D. V. (1984) Diagnostic implications of tear protein profiles. *Br. J. Ophthalmol.*, **68**, 321–324.

Manthorpe, R. *et al.* (1986) The Copenhagen criteria for Sjögren's syndrome. *Scand. J. Rheumatol.*, **61(Suppl.)**, 19–21.

Marquardt, R. and Wenz, F. H. (1980) Investigations of the stability of the tear film. *Klin. Mbl. Augenheilk.*, **176**, 879–884.

Mathers, W. D., Laing, J. A. and Zimmerman, M. B. (1996a) Tear film changes associated with normal ageing. *Cornea*, **15**, 229–334.

Mathers, W. D. *et al.* (1996b) Model for ocular tear film function. *Cornea*, **15**, 110–119.

Maurice, D. (1973) Dynamics and drainage of tears. *Int. Ophthalmol. Clin.*, **13**, 103–114.

McGill, J. *et al.* (1984) Normal tear protein profiles and age-related changes. *Br. J. Ophthalmol.*, **68**, 316–320.

Medsger, T. A. and Masi, A. T. (1985) Epidemiology of rheumatic diseases. In *Arthritis and Allied Conditions* (ed. D. J. McCarty), Philadelphia, Lee and Febiger, pp. 9–39.

Millodot, M. (1977) The influence of age on the sensitivity of the cornea. *Invest. Ophthalmol. Vis. Sci.*, **16**, 230–241.

Mishima, S. *et al.* (1966) Determination of tear volume and tear flow. *Invest. Ophthalmol. Vis. Sci.*, **5**, 264–275.

Nelson, J. D. (1995) Simultaneous evaluation of tear turnover and corneal epithelial permeability by fluorophotometry in normal subjects and patients with kerato-conjunctivitis sicca (KCS). *Trans. Am. Ophthalmol. Soc.*, **93**, 709–753.

Norn, M. (1965) Tear secretion in normal eyes. *Acta Ophthalmol.*, **43**, 567–573.

Norn, M. (1966) Tear secretion in diseased eyes. *Acta Ophthalmol.*, **44**, 25–32.

Norn, M. S. (1974) The external eye. In *Examination Methods*, Scriptor, Copenhagen, p. 119.

Norn, M. S. (1985) Meibomian orifices and Marx's line, studied by triple vital staining, *Acta Ophthalmol. (Copenh.)*, **63**, 698–700.

Norn, M. S. (1987) Expressibility of meibomian secretion. *Acta Ophthalmol.*, **65**, 137–142.

Patel, S. and Farrell, J. (1988) Age-related changes in pre-corneal tear film stability. *Optom. Vis. Sci.*, **66**, 175–178.

Pietsch, R. L. and Polman, M. E. (1973) Human tear lysosyme variables. *Arch. Ophthalmol.*, **90**, 94–96.

Polak, B. C. P. (1987) Side effects of drugs and tear function. *Doc. Ophthalmol.*, **67**, 115–119.

Port, M. and Asaria, T. (1990) The assessment of human tear volume. *J. Br. Cont. Lens Assoc.*, **13**, 77–82.

Records, R. E. (1979) Tear film. In *Physiology of the Eye and Visual System* (ed. R. E. Records), Hagerstown, Harper & Row, pp. 47–67.

Rolando, M. J. and Refojo, M. (1983) Tear evaporimeter for measuring water evaporation rate from the tear film under controlled conditions in humans. *Exp. Eye Res.*, **36**, 25–33.

Schein, O. D. *et al.* (1996) Estimating the prevalence of dry eye among elderly Americans: SEE project. *Invest. Ophthalmol. Vis. Sci.*, **37(3)**, S646.

Seal, D. V. *et al.* (1986) Bacteriology and tear protein profiles of the dry eye. *Br. J. Ophthalmol.*, **70**, 122–125.

Sen, D. K. and Sarin, G. S. (1980) Immuno-assay of human tear lysosyme. *Am. J. Ophthalmol.*, **90**, 715–718.

Sen, D. K. *et al.* (1976) Immunoglobulins in tears of normal Indian people. *Br. J. Ophthalmol.*, **60**, 302–304.

Shearn, M. A. (1971) Sjögren's syndrome. In *Major Problems, Internal Medicine* (ed. L. H. Smith, Jnr), Philadelphia, W. B. Saunders, Vol. II.

Stasior, O. G. and Roen, J. L. (1994) Thoughts on the ductiles of the ageing human lacrimal gland. *Adv. Exp. Med. Biol.*, **350**, 49–52.

Stiewe, M. (1962) Alternsabhangigkeit der Transensekretion. *Aternsforsch*, **15**, 318–323.

Strehler, B. L. (1962). *Time, Cells and Ageing*, New York, Academic Press.

Strickland, R. W. *et al.* (1987) The frequency of sicca syndrome in an elderly female population. *J. Rheumatol.*, **14**, 766–771.

Sullivan, D. A. *et al.* (1998a) Influence of gender and sex steroid hormones on the structure and function of the lacrimal gland. *Adv. Exp. Med. Biol.*, **438**, 11–42.

Sullivan, D. A. *et al.* (1998b) Androgen regulation of the meibomian gland. *Adv. Exp. Med. Biol.*, **438**, 327–332.

Tomlinson, A. (1992) *Complications of Contact Lens Wear*. St Louis, Mosby, p. 195.

Tomlinson, A. and Giesbrecht, C. (1993) The ageing tear film. *J. Br. Cont. Lens Assoc.*, **16**, 67–69.

Tomlinson, A., Craig, J. P. and Lowther, G. E. (1998) The biophysical role in tear regulation. In *Lacrimal Gland, Tear Film and Dry Eye Syndromes 2* (eds D. A. Sullivan *et al.*), *Adv. Exp. Med. Biol.*, **438**, 371–380.

Ungar, H. (1967) Diseases of ageing. In *Pathology* (ed. S. L. Robins), Philadelphia, W. B. Saunders, p. 502.

Vitali, C. *et al.* (1993) Preliminary criteria for the classification of Sjögren's syndrome. *Arthr. Rheum.*, **36**, 340–347.

Wright, J. C. and Mager, R. G. (1962) A review of the Schirmer test for tear production. *Arch. Ophthalmol.*, **67**, 564–565.

5 Pathology of the tear film

George Smith

Introduction

The presence of contact lenses can affect the integrity of the preocular tear film and any pre-existing abnormality of the tear film is likely to be exacerbated by contact lens wear. An appreciation of the causes of dry eye, current therapeutic options and possible future therapies is therefore of importance to the contact lens practitioner. It is also important to investigate some of the pathological processes influencing the integrity of the tear film.

The main functions of the preocular tear film are to maintain the corneal and conjunctival epithelium in its normal state and also to provide a smooth corneal refracting surface. The tear film acts as a lubricant and supplies oxygen, anti-infectious agents and reparative substances to the epithelial surfaces. If the tear film is abnormal, the ocular surface will also be affected.

Tear film abnormalities

There are two main reasons why the tear film may function inadequately; ineffective resurfacing, and inadequate quantity or quality of the tear components.

Ineffective resurfacing

For normal resurfacing to occur there must be a normal blink reflex, normal corneal epithelium and congruity between the external ocular surface and eyelids. Ineffective resurfacing can occur in any condition where the blink reflex is abnormal; neurological diseases which affect the seventh cranial nerve are a good example. In other conditions there may be a mechanical failure in the eyelid closing mechanism. This can occur as a result of scarring resulting in multiple symblepharon formation. Such scarring occurs commonly in ocular pemphigoid, erythema multiforme, Stevens-Johnson syndrome and chemical burns. In scarring disorders, as well as ineffective resurfacing there is often the problem of ingrowing eyelashes resulting in mechanical damage to the ocular surface.

In nocturnal lagophthalmos, drying of the cornea occurs at night as a result of an inability to keep the lids properly closed during sleep. Another variant of this is the so-called 'floppy eyelid' syndrome. This is an uncommon and a frequently misdiagnosed condition, which typically affects obese men in whom a rubbery tarsus and loose upper eyelid evert during sleep, exposing the upper tarsus and rendering the upper tarsal conjunctiva and cornea susceptible to trauma. Examination shows bilateral or unilateral chronic papillary conjunctivitis of the exposed tarsal conjunctiva. The upper lids are extremely loose and readily evert when elevated. Treatment involves protection of the eye during sleep with a shield or taping the lids shut to prevent lid eversion. A permanent cure can be achieved by horizontal lid shortening.

Abnormal eyelid apposition to the globe is a relatively common problem, especially in elderly patients. The ageing process leads to lid laxity that can result in either a turning in of the lid, as the preseptal orbicularis muscle overrides the pretarsal orbicularis resulting in an entropion, or inward rotation of the eyelid. This causes the eyelashes to rub on the cornea and produce symptoms of irritation. A similar process results in ectropion, where the eyelid turns outwards and poor lid apposition causes drying of the globe and keratinization of the exposed conjunctiva. Surgical correction of these disorders can result in normal function being restored.

In the worldwide setting, probably one of the most important causes of ocular irritation is upper lid entropion and misdirection of lashes as a result of scarring secondary to trachoma. Trachoma is still one of the most common causes of blindness in the world today and is caused by an infective organism, *Chlamydia trachomatis*. Chronic inflammation and reinfection results in scarring of the eyelids and eventually leads to painful upper lid entropion and corneal infections. Prevention is very important in this disorder, as once serious deformity has occurred it is very difficult to prevent corneal scarring and penetrating keratoplasty is unlikely to be successful. Leprosy is another condition that can result in eyelid abnormalities and corneal scarring and, like trachoma, is preventable if diagnosed early.

Ocular pemphigoid is seen quite commonly in corneal clinics in the developed world and can be disheartening to manage. It is an autoimmune disorder of unknown aetiology that results in relentless scarring of the conjunctiva. In progressive cases severe keratinization of the conjunctiva results in blindness as the cornea dries out and eventually becomes keratinized itself. In some cases the process can be halted or modified by the use of immunosuppressive agents and steroids, but in others the condition continues until the only remaining strategy is the insertion of a keratoprosthesis.

Inadequate quantity or quality of the tear components

These conditions may be categorized as follows:

- Aqueous deficiency, e.g. keratoconjunctivitis sicca
- Soluble surfactant (mucin) deficiency
- Lipid abnormalities (blepharitis and meibomian gland dysfunction).

Keratoconjunctivitis sicca

One of the problems in dealing with dry eye conditions is the lack of a precise definition. The term keratoconjunctivitis sicca (KCS) has been used loosely to describe dry eye disorders. In the United Kingdom, KCS tends to be used to describe the autoimmune destruction of the lacrimal gland, whereas in the United States the term is more loosely used to describe other dry eye disorders.

Because of the previous confusion associated with terminology in KCS, dry eye is a more appropriate term to use for classifying these disorders. One such classification divides dry eye into:

1. Tear-deficient dry eye:
   - Non-Sjögren's dry eye
   - Sjögren's dry eye.
2. Evaporative dry eye:
   - Blepharitis-associated – anterior and posterior blepharitis
   - Ocular mucin deficiencies
   - Blink disorders
   - Disorders of lid aperture and lid/globe congruity
   - Ocular surface disorders
   - Other tear film disorders (contact lens induced).

Dry eye can result from a malfunction of the lacrimal gland. Pure KCS is an autoimmune disorder affecting the lacrimal gland and resulting in atrophy and fibrosis of the gland tissue after the patient's own immune system has attacked it. The destruction of the lacrimal and salivary gland is secondary to lymphocytic infiltration. Neither the reason for lymphocytic infiltration nor the mechanism for acinar destruction is known. In this and other autoimmune diseases, research has focused on specialized functions of the immune cells and their products (e.g. cytokines).

Particular attention has centred on the interaction between MHC molecules and T-cell receptors and on specific autoantibodies and autoantigen interactions. This has led to a large body of information on immune repertoire, but offers few clues for treatment. Recent investigation into Sjögren's syndrome has focused more on generalized functions that the immune cells share with other cells. Chief among these is the important homeostatic mechanism called apoptosis, or programmed cell death. Apoptosis was of interest initially to embryologists studying cell deletion during foetal development. For example, apoptosis of foetal interdigital webs is responsible for the development of digits.

Many animal cells undergo apoptotic cell death when exposed to viruses. The cell, once aware of the virus, initiates its own suicide mechanism, blocking cellular production of additional viral particles. Fas/APO-1 is a transmembrane protein that mediates programmed cell death. The relationship between programmed cell death and autoimmunity first became apparent when a mutated Fas/APO-1 gene was found in genetically autoimmune susceptible mice.

The problem of lacrimal gland destruction in Sjögren's syndrome poses two questions in relation to lymphocyte biology:

1. What attracts immune cells to the site in the first place?
2. Once immune cells enter these target organs and commence the destructive process, why do they never leave?

Lymphocytes will diminish if steroids or immunosuppressive drugs are given to the patient. Left untreated, however, the process is relentless. The mechanism responsible for the attraction of lymphocytes into a target organ is unknown, but genetic, viral, and hormonal factors may all be involved. It is generally assumed that this process represents an immune response to a viral or autoantigen.

Research suggests that the cause of dryness in Sjögren's syndrome is due to apoptotic cell death of acinar epithelial cells. Salivary gland biopsies in patients suffering from this syndrome reveal that infiltrating lymphocytes are Fas positive, showing a commitment to apoptosis. The condition may soon be understood on the basis of inappropriate lymphocyte cell survival related to cytokine dysregulation and the function of oncogenes and autogenes. Cytokine therapy to restore autoregulatory balance could be an appropriate new treatment for immune-based dry eye syndromes.

More recently, attention has been focused by some researchers on the inflammatory mechanisms that may be involved in dry eye patients. They postulate a so-called 'final common pathway' or unified theory of dry eye. Under this theory, in postmenopausal women an androgen protective effect occurs and androgen levels are reduced. This is thought to render the lacrimal gland more susceptible to immunological damage from T cells and autoantibodies. If this theory proves to be correct, at least in a proportion of patients, it could result in the development of exciting new immunomodulatory compounds that may be beneficial in these patients and reduce further damage to the lacrimal gland. This represents a new approach to the problem and encourages further research into the development of novel compounds that may be more effective than our current therapies.

One exciting new compound is cyclosporine. This compound has been used successfully for nearly a decade in the treatment of canine KCS, prompting researchers to evaluate it for use in a number of human ocular autoimmune disorders. Results of the studies have established the efficacy of ophthalmic cyclosporine in a variety of conditions including KCS, vernal keratoconjunctivitis and ligneous conjunctivitis, as well as in corneal transplant patients.

The mechanism of action of cyclosporine in the treatment of KCS may be two-fold. Cyclosporine's primary mechanism of action is as an immune modulator that prevents T-cell mediated immunoreactivity. Patients with KCS have significantly increased numbers of cytokine-secreting T-cells in their conjunctiva. These cytokines may be responsible for localized inflammation and irritation associated with KCS. Cyclosporine has a local immunoregulatory effect on the conjunctiva and is most likely mediated through the local suppression of the T-cell population. In addition, cyclosporine may act as a lacrimomimetic agent. Based on observational reports of post-transplant patients, the effect of cyclosporine on tear production was evaluated in a cohort of patients before and after kidney transplantation. All patients received oral cyclosporine following the transplant procedure to prevent organ rejection. Tear production was increased significantly following transplantation, as compared to pre-transplant/pre-cyclosporine levels.

Recently, other researchers have postulated that a decrease in oestrogen levels over a long period of time results in changes to the conjunctival epithelium that may render it susceptible to inflammatory changes such as in atrophic vaginitis. One study showed that topically applied oestradiol improved symptoms and increased tear secretion in dry eye patients as measured by the Schirmer test.

Sometimes dry eye is part of a more generalized autoimmune disorder. Dry eye is classified as Sjögren's syndrome in the presence of hypergammaglobulinaemia (50 per cent of cases), rheumatoid arthritis (70–90 per cent of cases), and antinuclear antibody (up to 80 per cent of cases). Involvement of the salivary glands causes a dry mouth and other mucous membranes such as the bronchial epithelium and vagina may also be affected. When these features occur in isolation, the disorder is termed a primary Sjögren's syndrome. When they are associated with a generalized connective tissue disorder, the condition is classified as secondary Sjögren's syndrome. Other systemic associations of secondary Sjögren's syndrome include systemic lupus erythematosis, systemic sclerosis, psoriatic arthritis, juvenile chronic arthritis, polymyositis, Hashimoto's thyroiditis, and primary biliary cirrhosis. The presence of rheumatoid arthritis can cause the additional problem of hand and finger deformities that can make the administration of drops difficult. The manufacturers of dry eye preparations should keep this in mind when preparing packaging.

Miscellaneous causes of non-Sjögren's KCS include the following:

- Destruction of lacrimal tissue by tumours, sarcoidosis or chronic inflammation (pseudotumour, dysthyroid ophthalmopathy). Graft versus host disease, HIV infection and dacryoadenitis are other conditions that can damage the lacrimal gland
- Meibomian gland dysfunction, which destabilizes the tear film
- Absence of the lacrimal gland, either following its surgical removal for tumour or, more rarely, congenital
- Blockage of the excretory ducts of the lacrimal gland as a result of severe conjunctival scarring, which may also cause mucin deficiency through destruction of the goblet cells
- Neurological lesions such as familial dysautonomia (Riley–Day syndrome)
- Reflex hyposecretion, as in neuroparalytic keratitis, chronic contact lens wear and proximal seventh cranial nerve palsy
- Uncertain category situations, such as multiple neuromatosis and *cri du chat* syndrome.

Clinical evaluation

Symptoms

The most common symptoms of KCS are irritation, a foreign-body sensation, burning, the presence of stringy mucous discharge and transient blurring of vision. Less frequent symptoms include itching, photophobia and a tired or heavy feeling to the eyelids. Patients with severe filamentary keratitis may complain of severe pain brought on by blinking. Surprisingly, patients seldom complain that their eyes are dry, although some may report a lack of emotional tears or a deficient response when peeling onions. The symptoms of KCS are frequently exacerbated by exposure to conditions associated with increased tear evaporation (e.g. air conditioning, wind) or on prolonged reading when the blink reflex is reduced. Closing the eyes may reduce the symptoms. The diagnosis of dry eye cannot, however, be made on symptoms alone, since most of these can be caused by other conditions. It is vitally important, therefore, that the symptoms are taken in context with the clinical features and the results of tests of tear function.

Clinical features

Tear film abnormalities

The following tear film abnormalities are characteristic of KCS:

- An increase in mucous strands and debris is an early sign. In the normal eye, as the tear film breaks down the mucin layer becomes contaminated with lipid but is washed away. In the dry eye, the lipid-contaminated mucin accumulates in the tear film and tends to move with each blink. Mucin also has the interesting property of drying very quickly and rehydrating very slowly.
- The marginal tear meniscus is concave, small and in severe cases may be absent altogether. In normal eyes, the meniscus is convex and about 1 mm high.

Corneal abnormalities

Keratopathy of the following types may be seen in moderate to severe cases of KCS:

1. Punctate epitheliopathy involving the inferior cornea
2. Filaments consisting of small comma-shaped opacities with the unattached end hanging over the surface of the cornea and moving with each blink. Filaments stain readily with rose bengal (Figure 5.1)
3. Mucous plaques consisting of semi-transparent, white-to-grey, slightly elevated lesions of various sizes and shapes. The plaques are composed of mucus, epithelial cells, and proteinaceous and lipoidal material. They are usually seen in association with corneal filaments and also stain with rose bengal.

Special tests

In clinical practice there is no one test of tear function that enables the clinician to make a definitive diagnosis of dry eye. The clinician therefore has to rely on a combination of different tests and also his or her clinical experience. In some cases it is obvious that the patient has poor tear function, but in others it may be more difficult to make the correct

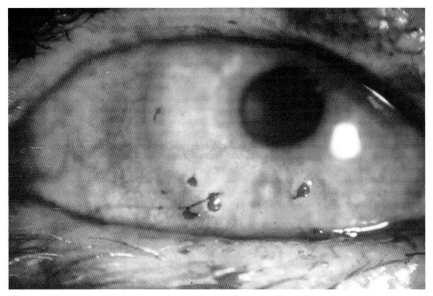

Figure 5.1 Filaments stain readily with rose bengal (from Kanski, 1994, with permission)

diagnosis. Lid margin disease is very common in the general population and is an important cause of tear film instability.

Tear film break-up time

Measurement of tear film break-up time (BUT) assesses precorneal tear film stability. It is performed as follows:

1. Fluorescein is instilled into the lower fornix
2. The patient is asked to blink several times and then stop
3. The tear film is examined with a broad beam and a cobalt blue filter. After an interval of time, black spots or lines indicating the formation of dry areas will appear.

The BUT is the interval between the last blink and the appearance of the first randomly distributed dry spot. The development of dry spots always in the same location should be ignored because this is caused by a local corneal surface abnormality and not by an intrinsic instability of the tear film. A BUT of less than 10 s is abnormal.

Rose bengal staining

Rose bengal is a dye with an affinity for dead and devitalized epithelial cells and mucus. The typical staining pattern in KCS consists of two triangles with their bases at the limbus. Corneal filaments and plaques are also shown up more clearly by the dye. One disadvantage of rose bengal is that it may cause ocular irritation, which can last for up to a day, particularly in severely dry eyes. In order to reduce the amount of irritation, a very small drop should be used but topical anaesthetic should not be instilled before staining because it may induce a false-positive result. Attempts to quantify rose bengal staining patterns have been made by giving a score to the degree of stain observed.

Rose bengal staining is very useful in differentiating dry eye disorders from another condition, known as a superior limbic keratoconjunctivitis (SLK). This is an uncommon, chronic, inflammatory disorder, that typically affects middle-aged women. Between 20 and 50 per cent of patients have associated thyroid disease. The condition is frequently misdiagnosed because symptoms are more severe than clinical findings would suggest.

Clinical features

SLK is usually bilateral, although the severity of involvement may be asymmetrical. The course is prolonged, with remissions and exacerbations until eventual resolution occurs without sequelae. Presentation is with non-specific symptoms of a foreign-body sensation, burning, photophobia and mucous discharge. Examination of the superior conjunctiva and cornea shows the following:

- Papillary hypertrophy of the superior tarsus, which may give rise to diffuse velvety appearance
- Hyperaemia of the superior bulbar conjunctiva, which is most intense at the limbus and fades as it approaches the superior fornix; the epithelial cells may be keratinized and the affected area may lack lustre
- Papillary hypertrophy at the limbus
- Punctate epithelial erosions at the superior cornea are common
- Corneal filaments occur in about one-third of cases and are not necessarily associated with diminished tear secretion
- KCS is present in about 25 per cent of cases.

Treatment

Treatment of SLK is aimed primarily at altering the abnormal mechanical interaction between the upper eyelid and the superior corneal limbus. Although there is no definitive treatment, the following therapeutic options are available:

- Topical medication with a 1 per cent adrenaline drops may give symptomatic relief in mild cases. The number of corneal filaments can be reduced with 5 per cent acetylcystine drops. Patients with associated KCS should have tear substitutes.
- Soft contact lenses are useful in some patients.
- Thermocauterization of the superior bulbar conjunctiva appears to be safe and effective in a high proportion of cases.
- Resection of the superior limbal conjunctiva may help in resistant cases.
- Correction of thyroid dysfunction, if present, is also beneficial.

The Schirmer test

The Schirmer test (Figure 5.2) is useful when slit-lamp signs of KCS are absent yet the presence of the condition is suspected. The test is performed by measuring the amount of wetting of a special (Whatman) filter paper, which is 5 mm wide and 35 mm long. It can be performed with or without prior instillation of a topical anaesthetic. In theory, when performed without an anaesthetic the test measures total secretion (i.e. basic and reflex), whereas with an anaesthetic it measures only basic secretion. In practice, however, although topical anaesthesia reduces the amount of reflex secretion it does not eliminate it completely. The test is performed as follows:

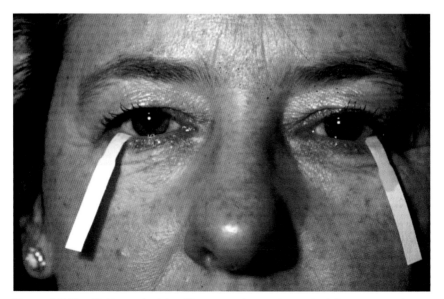

Figure 5.2 The Schirmer test is still commonly used as a test for aqueous tear production (from Kanski, 1994, with permission)

1. The eye is gently dried with tissue paper over closed lids to mop up any excess secretion
2. The filter paper is folded 5 mm from one end and inserted at the junction of the middle and outer third of the lower lid
3. The patient is asked to keep the eyes open and to blink as necessary
4. After 5 minutes the filter paper is removed and the amount of wetting is measured.

A normal result is over 15 mm without topical anaesthesia and slightly less with anaesthesia. Between 5–10 mm is borderline and less than 5 mm indicates impaired secretion. Some authorities suggest that the cut-off point between normal and abnormal is 6 mm. It is important to note whether local anaesthesia has been used or not, as repeated testing should be done under conditions that are as similar as possible.

Phenol red thread test
In the phenol red test, a strip of cotton is inserted into the lower fornix (nasal side) for 15 s. The amount of colour change is measured in mm. This test has an advantage over the Schirmer test in that it produces less foreign-body sensation and stimulates less reflex secretion. In time, this technique may supersede the Schirmer test.

Tear osmolarity
In KCS the tears tend to be of hyperosmolar consistency. Measuring the osmolarity of the tears has therefore been used to assess aqueous tear deficiency. In fact measuring osmolarity is perhaps the most reliable test for tear function, as most dry eye states have been shown to exhibit hyperosmolarity. The problem lies in the absence of an accurate and easily applied test to measure tear osmolarity. Hopefully, a commercially available test will be developed. This, combined with serological tests to differentiate autoimmune from non-autoimmune dry eye disorders, will herald a new era in the diagnosis and management of these conditions.

Lysozyme assays
There is evidence to suggest that the lysozyme content in tears decreases in KCS and that this effect parallels the decrease in aqueous tear production. Because of this finding, it has been stated that measuring the lysozyme in tears represents an accurate diagnostic test for KCS. However, lysozyme assays have not gained popularity as they are cumbersome to perform and need to be carried out by a laboratory which is set up to conduct such tests on a routine basis. Facilities are required for filter paper electrophoresis, for the maintenance of a strain of bacteria (*Micrococcus lysodiekticus*) and for assessing the inhibition of different dilutions of tears on bacterial growth.

Symptomatic treatment

The main aims of treatment of dry eye are to relieve discomfort, provide a smooth optical surface and prevent structural corneal damage. In general, once a diagnosis of dry eye has been made, the patient should be discouraged from wearing his or her contact lenses while the treatment is being carried out. If the condition is later deemed to be a minor case of tear film instability related to blepharitis or only minor tear deficiency, then judicial use of the contact lenses can be re-introduced. It should be remembered that the wearing of contact lenses may interfere with the treatment and that an already compromised tear film is more prone to infection in the presence of contact lenses. One or more of the following measures may be used simultaneously.

Preservation of existing tears

- Reduction of room temperature (or avoiding a warm room with central heating) may be helpful since this causes increased evaporation of tears
- Room humidifiers may be used but are frequently disappointing because the apparatus is incapable of significantly increasing the relative humidity of an average sized room; however, a temporary local increase in humidity can be achieved with moist chamber goggles
- A small lateral tarsorrhaphy can be performed, since decreasing the surface area of the interpalpebral fissure may be helpful in patients with incomplete lid closure.

Topical treatment

Tear substitutes
Tear substitutes (artificial tears) form the mainstay of treatment of mild to moderate KCS. It is crucial that the patient uses the drops frequently and regularly; in severe cases they must be instilled at half-hourly or hourly intervals, whereas in milder cases use four times a day may suffice. The main disadvantages of drops are short duration and the development of sensitivity to the preservative, although the latter can be avoided by using preservative-free units (Minims).

The three main groups of eye drop tear substitutes are:

1. Cellulose derivatives
2. Polyvinyl alcohol
3. Mucomimetics.

In theory, mucomimetics create a stable hydrophilic corneal surface and enhance corneal wetting, but in practice they do not appear to be superior to the other types of preparation. For this reason, the patient must select the most suitable and least irritating preparation by trial and error. Ointments containing petrolatum mineral oil (Lacrilube™) can be used at bedtime.

Mucolytic agents

Five per cent acetylcysteine drops may be useful in patients with corneal filaments and mucous plaques. The drops are used four times daily and may cause some irritation following instillation. Acetylcysteine is also malodorous and has a limited bottle life so that its use is limited to two weeks.

Reduction of tear drainage

Punctal occlusion preserves the natural tears and prolongs the effect of artificial tears. It is of greatest value in patients with severe KCS, particularly when associated with toxicity from preservatives. Occlusion may be temporary or permanent.

Temporary punctal occlusion

Short-term occlusion of the puncta can be achieved by inserting into the canaliculi either a commercially available plug or silicone rod, or a 2/0 catgut suture. The main aim of temporary occlusion is to ensure that epiphora does not occur following permanent occlusion. Initially, all four puncta are occluded and the patient is reviewed after one week. If epiphora is induced, the upper plugs are removed and the patient is re-examined one week later. If the patient is now asymptomatic, the plugs are removed and the inferior canaliculi are permanently occluded.

Temporary punctal plugs have also been used by some authorities to enable patients who have slightly dry eyes to continue wearing their contact lenses. In this situation silicon plugs can be used to good effect; however, great care should be taken when allowing patients with dry eye to continue wearing contact lenses as the risk of infection in these patients is increased. Such patients should also be checked regularly to make sure that the silicon plugs are not causing irritation.

Permanent punctal occlusion

Permanent punctual occlusion (Figure 5.3) should be undertaken only in patients with severe KCS and repeated Schirmer test values of 2 mm or less. It should not be performed in patients who develop epiphora following temporary occlusion of only the inferior puncta. Permanent occlusion should also be avoided in young patients, whose tear production tends to fluctuate. Occlusion is achieved by first dilating the punctum vigorously and then gently heating the mucosal lining of the proximal canaliculus for 1 s with cautery and black heat. Following

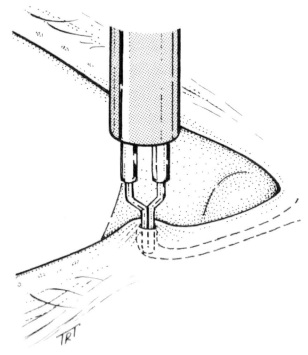

Figure 5.3 Permanent punctal cautery is achieved by thermal damage to the puncti (from Kanski, 1994, with permission)

successful punctal occlusion, it is important to watch for signs of recanalization. Argon laser canaliculoplasty is another method of occlusion, which is not as effective in the long term as cauterization. It is also important in these cases to treat any associated disorder such as chronic blepharitis.

Chronic blepharitis

Chronic blepharitis (Figure 5.4) is an inflammation of the lid margins. It is a very common external eye disorder, the exact aetiology of which is unclear, although staphylococcal infection and seborrhoea play important roles. The management of chronic blepharitis is frequently unsatisfactory because there is no definitive treatment. As a result of the intimate relationship between the lids and ocular surface, chronic blepharitis may also cause secondary changes in the conjunctiva and cornea, and many patients have associated tear film instability. Apart from causing

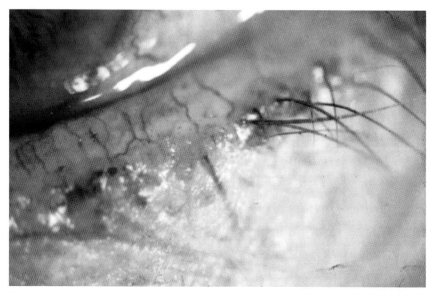

Figure 5.4 Chronic anterior blepharitis (from Kanski, 1994, with permission)

annoying symptoms, the condition may also interfere with contact lens wear and aggravate treatment of patients with dry eye.

The two main types of chronic blepharitis are anterior and posterior. Anterior blepharitis refers to dysfunction of the glands of Zeis and Moll and also to staphylococcal infection of the lash follicles. Posterior blepharitis, on the other hand, refers to dysfunction of the meibomian glands. Although for descriptive purposes it is useful to separate anterior from posterior blepharitis, in clinical practice there is often an overlap between the two conditions. The symptoms of the various types of blepharitis are similar, although there is frequently little correlation between their severity and the extent of clinical involvement. Many of the symptoms are caused by secondary tear film instability. The most common symptoms are burning, a foreign-body sensation, mild photophobia and lid crusting, which are frequently worse in the mornings and are characterized by remissions and exacerbations.

Staphylococcal anterior blepharitis

Staphylococcal blepharitis is caused by chronic infection of the bases of the lashes that results in the formation of tiny intrafollicular abscesses. This leads to secondary dermal and epidermal ulceration and tissue destruction. Staphylococcal blepharitis is frequently seen in patients with atopic eczema and is more common in females than males. It tends to affect younger patients than seborrhoeic blepharitis and may start in childhood.

Clinical features

Examination of the anterior lid margins reveals hyperaemia, telangiectasis and scaling. The scales are hard and brittle and tend to be centred around the bases of the lashes (collarettes). When removed they may leave behind a tiny bleeding ulcer. Involvement of the lashes is greater in staphylococcal than in seborrhoeic blepharitis. In severe cases the lashes may become matted with yellow crust.

Complications in severe long-standing cases include trichiasis, madarosis (loss of lashes) and occasionally poliosis (white lashes). The anterior lid margin may become scarred, notched and hypertrophic. Spread of the infection to the glands of Zeis or Moll may give rise to an acute external hordeolum (stye) and involvement of the meibomian glands can lead to an internal hordeolum. Recurrent attacks of acute bacterial conjunctivitis may also occur.

Secondary changes caused by hypersensitivity to staphylococcal exotoxins include the following:

- Mild papillary conjunctivitis
- Toxic punctate epitheliopathy, primarily involving the inferior third of the cornea
- Marginal keratitis (catarrhal ulcer)
- Rarely, phlyctenulosis and pannus formation
- Associated tear film instability, seen in about 50 per cent of cases.

Treatment

Crucial to the treatment of blepharitis is the patient's motivation and ability to comply with instructions. The patient should be informed that complete eradication may not be possible but elimination of symptoms is usually effective. In severe and very long-standing cases, several weeks of intensive treatment may be necessary to achieve improvement.

The following strategies may be used:

1. Lid hygiene is the mainstay of treatment. It is aimed at removing crusts and toxic products by scrubbing the lid margins twice daily with either a commercially available lid scrub or a cotton bud dipped in a 25 per cent solution of baby shampoo. Alternatively, a face cloth or

handkerchief can be used. It is also useful to scrub the eyelids when washing the hair. Gradually, lid hygiene can be performed less frequently as the condition is brought under control.

2. Antibiotic ointment such as bacitracin or erythromycin should be rubbed into the anterior lid margins with a clean finger after all crusts have been removed. Ideally, the organisms should be identified and their sensitivity to various antibiotics tested.

3. Weak topical steroids such as fluoromethalone and clobetasone used four times daily for a few days are useful for secondary papillary conjunctivitis, toxic epitheliopathy, marginal keratitis and phlyctenulosis.

4. Artificial tears for associated tear film instability are required in about 50 per cent of cases. Unless this aspect of the disease is recognized and treated, relief of symptoms will be incomplete. During the first 1–2 weeks the drops should be used frequently.

Seborrhoeic anterior blepharitis

Seborrhoeic blepharitis (Figure 5.5) is a disorder of the glands of Zeis and Moll and is frequently associated with seborrhoeic dermatitis. The seborrhoeic skin changes may involve the scalp, eyebrows, nasolabial folds, retroauricular areas and sternum. The two main forms of seborrhoeic blepharitis are the oily type, in which the scaly eruptions are greasy, and the dry type (pityriasis capitis or dandruff). It has been postulated that the excessive amounts of neutral lipids in patients with seborrhoeic dermatitis are broken down by a bacterial lipase into irritating fatty acids.

This form of blepharitis may occur in isolation, or it may be associated with staphylococcal or posterior blepharitis. The symptoms of pure seborrhoeic blepharitis are similar to but less severe than those in staphylococcal blepharitis, with fewer remissions and exacerbations. About 30 per cent of patients have associated tear film instability.

Clinical features

Examination of the anterior lid margins shows a shiny telangiectasis. There is dandruff-like desquamation of the epidermis that gives rise to yellow, greasy scales located anywhere on the lid margin. The scales are soft and do not leave a small ulcer when removed. The lashes are also greasy and stuck together. Secondary changes, which are uncommon and less severe than in staphylococcal blepharitis, are papillary conjunctivitis and punctate epitheliopathy involving mainly the middle third of the cornea.

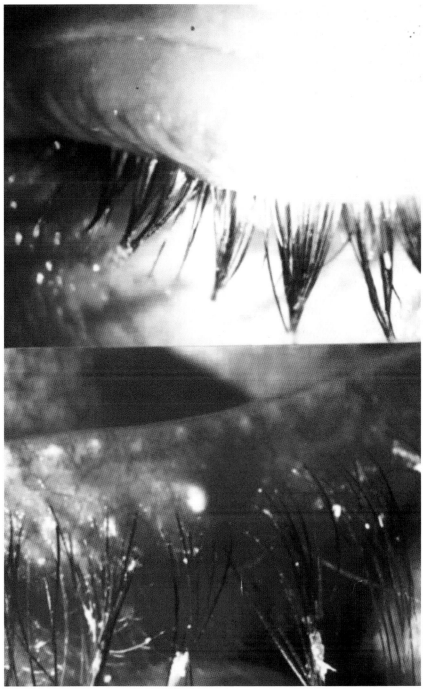

Figure 5.5 Seborrhoeic anterior blepharitis (from Kanski, 1994, with permission)

Treatment of pure seborrhoeic blepharitis is mainly with lid hygiene using bicarbonate of soda as a de-greasing agent. If necessary, artificial tears should also be used.

Posterior blepharitis

Posterior blepharitis (Figure 5.6) is caused by dysfunction of the meibomian glands. The condition may occur in isolation in the form of meibomian seborrhoea and primary meibomianitis, or more commonly it occurs in combination with seborrhoeic blepharitis, in which there is more generalized sebaceous gland abnormality.

Clinical features

The clinical features of posterior blepharitis vary from hypersecretion to gland stagnation and from patchy to diffuse meibomian gland involvement. The three main types are:

1. Meibomian seborrhoea
2. Primary meibomitis
3. Meibomitis with secondary blepharitis.

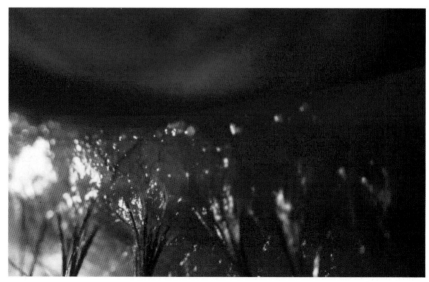

Figure 5.6 Posterior blepharitis (from Kanski, 1994, with permission)

Meibomian seborrhoea

Meibomian seborrhoea is characterized by dilated meibomian glands which are easily expressed to produce copious amounts of lipid. This appears on the lid margin as small oil globules or as collections of wax material. The tear film is excessively oily and foamy. In severe cases, the secretions accumulate as a frothy discharge at the inner canthi (meibomian foam). This type of posterior blepharitis is easy to miss because although the symptoms (burning sensation on first waking) may be severe, there are few, if any, signs of inflammatory lid disease.

Primary meibomitis

Primary meibomitis is characterized by diffuse inflammation centred around the meibomian gland orifices. Two-thirds of patients have associated acne rosacea and the remainder have seborrhoeic dermatitis. The following are the main clinical features:

- The meibomian gland orifices may show pouting and be capped by domes of oil (meibomana). The expressed meibomian gland secretions may be turbid and contain particulate matter. In advanced cases, firm pressure on the tarsal glands shows inspissated secretions as semi-solid plaques with a toothpaste-like consistency.
- Obliteration of the meibomian ducts may cause secondary cystic dilation and the formation of meibomian cysts. In advanced cases, the posterior lid margins may show thickening, rounding, vascularization and notching.
- Frequent secondary changes include papillary conjunctivitis and inferior punctate epitheliopathy. About 30 per cent of patients have associated tear film instability.

Meibomitis with secondary blepharitis

Meibomitis with secondary blepharitis is always associated with seborrhoeic dermatitis. In contrast to primary meibomitis, involvement of the meibomian glands is mild and patchy. The structures surrounding the glands are inflamed and the secretions are solidified and difficult to express. Secondary conjunctival and corneal changes are usually mild. About 25 per cent of patients have associated tear film instability.

Treatment

Systemic antibiotics are the mainstay of therapy. It is thought that they exert their effect by inhibiting the production of bacterial lipase and free fatty acids. The following antibiotics may be used:

- Tetracycline 250 mg twice daily for at least 1 month; the main contraindications to tetracycline are pregnancy, lactation and children under the age of 12 years
- Doxycycline 100 mg daily is a good alternative to tetracycline; it has fewer gastrointestinal side-effects and needs to be taken less frequently, and has the same contraindications as tetracycline
- Erythromycin is sometimes used when tetracycline or doxycycline is contraindicated, but its efficacy in the treatment of posterior blepharitis is not well established.

Other measures, including lid hygiene, topical steroids and artificial tears, are similar to those for anterior blepharitis. Warm compresses to melt solidified sebum and mechanical expression of the meibomian glands may reduce the amount of irritating lipids within the glands.

Psychological aspects of chronic irritation in conjunction with blepharitis are worthy of consideration. There are certainly some patients who develop an obsessional neurosis about their eyes and it is also clear that in such cases the degree of abnormality is far less than expected from the severity of symptoms reported. After a trial of therapy for blepharitis, such patients should be considered for psychological management of their condition, which may include antidepressants or psychotherapy. It should be remembered, however, that some antidepressants may adversely affect the production of tears.

Summary

The study of dry eye, which at first sight may appear to be an uninteresting topic, is now becoming a subject for further research. In the future, once dry eye disorders are better understood and more accurate tests exist to differentiate the different categories of the disease, new therapeutic approaches will be developed. These new therapies will be more precise in nature and designed to have an impact on the basic pathology rather than treating the problem symptomatically.

Further reading

Akramian, J., Wedrich, A., Nepp, J. and Sator, M. (1998) Estrogen therapy in keratoconjunctivitis sicca. In *Lacrimal Gland, Tear Film, and Dry Eye Syndromes 2* (eds Sullivan *et al.*), New York, Plenum Press.

Kanski, J. J. (1994) *Clinical Ophthalmology*, 3rd edn. Oxford, Butterworth-Heinemann, Chapter 4.

Lemp, M. A. (1987) *Duane's Clinical Ophthalmology.* Philadelphia, Harper & Row, Vol. 4, Chapter 14.

Lemp, M. A. (1995) Report of the National Eye Institute/Industry Workshop on Clinical Trials in Dry Eyes. *CLAO. J.,* **21(4)**, 221–232.

Talal, N., Nakabayashi, T., Letterio, J. *et al.* (1998) Cytokines may prove useful in the treatment of Sjögren's syndrome (SS) dry eye. In *Lacrimal Gland, Tear Film, and Dry Eye Syndromes 2* (eds Sullivan *et al.*), New York, Plenum Press.

Tauber, J. (1998) A dose-ranging clinical trial to assess the safety and efficacy of cyclosporine ophthalmic emulsion in patients with keratoconjuctivitis sicca. In *Lacrimal Gland, Tear Film, and Dry Eye Syndromes 2* (eds Sullivan *et al.*), New York, Plenum Press.

6 The tear film – its role today and in the future

Donald R. Korb

Introduction

The contributors to this text have presented a comprehensive review of contemporary knowledge of the tear film including its structure and function, its relationship to the conjunctiva and the cornea, the diagnostic examination of the tear film, the ageing of the tear film, and the pathological tear film and its treatment.

The number of diagnostic tests for the evaluation of tear film disorders and ocular surface compromise can appear overwhelming to the non-research based clinician. Further complicating tear film diagnosis are questions and controversies regarding many of the diagnostic tests. The evidence is conclusive that multiple tests of different types must be performed in order first to diagnose whether there is a tear film disorder and, if present, its probable cause. The clinician must decide which tests to use routinely, which tests to have available for further investigation, and the specific method of conducting each test. It is also important that the tests are carried out in correct sequence to prevent one test from interfering with the other (Bron, 1997).

This chapter provides an overview of the specific tests for the evaluation and diagnosis of the tear film and dry eye disorders that the non-research based clinician might use in everyday clinical practice, the questions and controversies regarding the diagnostic tests, and a strategy for their use.

Survey of 68 practitioners for preferred diagnostic tests

In considering the question of which tests should be used in everyday clinical practice, and when discussing this issue with a number of colleagues, I became aware of significant differences of opinion regarding which tests should be employed. It also became obvious, as pointed out by Pflugfelder (1996), that 'for years, there has been considerable confusion regarding the classification of dry eye conditions and the specificity of diagnostic tests for dry eye.' I therefore decided to seek the opinions of practising optometrists and ophthalmologists in the United States and throughout the world. The majority of these practitioners are recognized nationally and internationally and would be considered knowledgeable in the area of the tear film either by virtue of their publications, their status as diplomates in the Cornea and Contact Lens Section of the American Academy of Optometry, or their being ophthalmologists with additional qualifications in the area of the cornea/tear film.

A printed survey form was utilized with two questions: 'If you could use only one test for diagnosis of the tear film and dry eye, what would that test be?' and 'What would your second, third, and fourth choices be?' The survey also provided space for comments. The form did not mention any test or offer any other instructions. Although this type of questioning is subject to obvious criticism, it was designed to determine whether there was a consensus of a first choice test, or an armamentarium of tests, utilized by practitioners with special qualifications in this area.

The survey was conducted among 36 optometrists and 41 ophthalmologists from the United States, Canada, United Kingdom, Switzerland, Italy, Australia, and Japan. The respondents are listed by country and profession in tabular form. Responses were received from 34 optometrists (ODs) and 34 ophthalmologists (MDs) as follows:

	OD	MD
United States	26	28
Canada	2	0
United Kingdom	2	4
Switzerland	1	0
Italy	0	1
Australia	3	0
Japan	0	1

Frequency and use of preferred tests

The results of this survey revealed that no one single test was a dominant first choice of the majority of the respondents in either profession. This finding confirms the observation of Mathers et al. (1996) who stated: 'There is as yet no single test that completely evaluates the ocular tear film. Each test alone examines part of the process but does not explain the entire sufficiently. It is only when these tests are seen together that we get a more complete look at this dynamic process.'

In response to the question of their test of choice if only one test were allowed, the most frequent answer was history and/or dry eye questionnaire by 28 per cent of respondents. However, history would have unquestionably scored even higher if the survey had stated that history was a 'test'. Almost half of those reporting history as their first choice commented on whether history was considered a test. Thus, the 28 per cent of respondents who reported that history was their first choice test is particularly impressive. The second most frequent first choice test was fluorescein break-up time (FBUT), cited by 19 per cent of respondents; the third was fluorescein staining (including fluorescein sequential staining) by 13 per cent; and the fourth was rose bengal by 10 per cent. Four respondents reported using tear film osmolarity as a first or second choice; however, an additional seven commented that if the test were more clinically applicable they would use it as their first choice test.

The test most frequently included as one of the four choices was the Schirmer test and its modifications, which was used by 62 per cent of respondents (although it was the first choice of only 9 per cent). The second and third most frequent tests of the four choices were rose bengal staining and FBUT by 50 per cent, the fourth was fluorescein staining (including fluorescein sequential staining) by 48 per cent, and the fifth was history by 37 per cent.

There were the following differences in the frequency of use of tests by category of OD or MD:

1. The Schirmer test was used more frequently by MDs than ODs (79 per cent/44 per cent), and was the first choice of 18 per cent of MDs, as compared to 0 per cent of ODs
2. The phenol red test was used primarily by ODs and rarely by MDs (29 per cent/6 per cent)
3. Rose bengal staining was used more frequently by MDs than ODs (59 per cent/41 per cent)
4. FBUT was used slightly more by ODs (53 per cent/47 per cent)
5. Fluorescein staining (including fluorescein sequential staining) was used equally by MDs and ODs (50 per cent/47 per cent)
6. History was used more frequently by ODs (50 per cent/24 per cent); however, the semantic difficulty may have influenced the result
7. Meibomian gland evaluation was used infrequently by both groups (9 per cent for MDs/12 per cent for ODs)
8. Lipid layer evaluation was used infrequently by both groups (9 per cent for MDs/15 per cent for ODs).

Results are presented in Tables 6.1, 6.2, and 6.3.

Table 6.1 Rank order of preference for tear film diagnostic tests ($n = 68$ respondents)

Diagnostic tests	Rank order of preference				Total
	#1	#2	#3	#4	
Schirmer	6	12	6	13	37
Schirmer-modified	0	2	1	2	5
Phenol red test (Zone-Quick)	0	2	7	3	12
Fluorescein break-up time (FBUT)	13	6	10	5	34
Fluorescein staining	6	11	7	4	28
Fluorescein sequential staining	3	1	0	1	5
Rose bengal staining	7	8	11	8	34
Lissamine green	2	6	2	1	11
Fluorescein/rose bengal 'mixture'	1	0	0	0	1
Meibomian gland evaluation	0	1	3	3	7
Lipid layer evaluation	0	0	3	5	8
NIBUT	0	2	1	0	3
Meniscus height	2	5	8	1	16
Fluorescein clearance or tear dilution	2	0	0	1	3
Tear film osmolality	1	3	0	0	4
Tear lactoferrin	0	0	1	1	2
History	19	2	1	3	25
Slit-lamp examination	5	5	3	0	13
Particulate matter in tear film	1	2	0	0	3
Lysozyme	0	0	0	1	1
Conjunctival folds	0	0	1	0	1
Punctal plugs	0	0	0	1	1
Other*	0	0	3	4	7

*Other = rosacea, blink pattern, ocular sensitivity, aqueous layer thickness, Schirmer's fluorophotometric tear flow and volume, tear ferning, evaporative measurements.

Forty-nine per cent of respondents reported using four tests, 16 per cent reported the use of only three, while 25 per cent reported the use of 5–10 tests in the diagnosis of the dry eye. Not one respondent reported the use of only one or two tests. Rather, 15 per cent of all respondents specifically commented that it was important to conduct a comprehensive evaluation with multiple tests, since the causes of tear film disorders are multi-factorial. It is clear from this survey and the additional comments of the respondents that there is no one test that is adequate to diagnose disorders of the tear film.

The results of the survey support the 'global definition' of dry eye disorders as developed by the National Eye Institute/industry workshop on clinical trials in dry eyes (Lemp, 1995):

Table 6.2 Rank order of preference for tear film diagnostic tests (n = 34 MDs)

Diagnostic tests	Rank order of preference				Total
	#1	#2	#3	#4	
Schirmer	6	8	4	6	24
Schirmer-modified	0	2	1	0	3
Phenol red test (Zone-Quick)	0	0	1	1	2
Fluorescein break-up time (FBUT)	3	3	7	3	16
Fluorescein staining	4	4	6	2	16
Fluorescein sequential staining	1	0	0	0	1
Rose bengal staining	5	5	4	6	20
Lissamine green	2	3	1	1	7
Fluorescein/rose bengal 'mixture'	0	0	0	0	0
Meibomian gland evaluation	0	0	3	0	3
Lipid layer evaluation	0	0	0	3	3
NIBUT	0	0	0	0	0
Meniscus height	1	1	2	1	5
Fluorescein clearance or tear dilution	2	0	0	1	3
Tear film osmolality	0	3	0	0	3
Tear lactoferrin	0	0	0	0	0
History	6	0	0	2	8
Slit-lamp examination	3	4	3	0	10
Particulate matter in tear film	1	1	0	0	2
Lysozyme	0	0	0	1	1
Conjunctival folds	0	0	0	0	0
Punctal plugs	0	0	0	0	0
Other*	0	0	2	3	5

*Other = rosacea, blink pattern, ocular sensitivity, aqueous layer thickness, Schirmer's fluorophotometric tear flow and volume, tear ferning, evaporative measurements.

Dry eye is a disorder of the tear film due to tear deficiency or excessive tear evaporation which causes damage to the inter-palpebral ocular surface and is associated with symptoms of ocular discomfort.

The three critical components required for defining the dry eye are:

1. Disorder of the tear film, due to tear deficiency or excessive tear evaporation
2. Damage to the interpalpebral ocular surface
3. Specific symptoms of ocular discomfort.

The first choices of the survey respondents were those tests which most readily and efficiently evaluated the three components of the definition:

**Table 6.3 Rank order of preference for tear film diagnostic tests
(*n* = 34 ODs)**

Diagnostic tests	Rank order of preference				Total
	#1	#2	#3	#4	
Schirmer	0	4	2	7	13
Schirmer-modified	0	0	0	2	2
Phenol red test (Zone-Quick)	0	2	6	2	10
Fluorescein break-up time (FBUT)	10	3	3	2	18
Fluorescein staining	2	7	1	2	12
Fluorescein sequential staining	2	1	0	1	4
Rose bengal staining	2	3	7	2	14
Lissamine green	0	3	1	0	4
Fluorescein/rose bengal 'mixture'	1	0	0	0	1
Meibomian gland evaluation	0	1	0	3	4
Lipid layer evaluation	0	0	3	2	5
NIBUT	0	2	1	0	3
Meniscus height	1	4	6	0	11
Fluorescein-clearance or tear dilution	0	0	0	0	0
Tear film osmolality	1	0	0	0	1
Tear lactoferrin	0	0	1	1	2
History	13	2	1	1	17
Slit-lamp examination	2	1	0	0	3
Particulate matter in tear film	0	1	0	0	1
Lysozyme	0	0	0	0	0
Conjunctival folds	0	0	1	0	1
Punctal plugs	0	0	0	1	1
Other*	0	0	1	1	2

*Other = rosacea, blink pattern, ocular sensitivity, aqueous layer thickness, Schirmer's
fluorophotometric tear flow and volume, tear ferning, evaporative measurements.

symptoms through history; surface disorders detected by fluorescein and
rose bengal staining; and tear deficiencies by the Schirmer test.

Summary of survey results

In summary, the survey revealed and/or confirmed the following:

- There is no one single test that is adequate for contemporary
  diagnosis of all tear film disorders
- Multiple tests are required to diagnose the nature of the tear film
  disorder
- History is the most frequent first choice test (28 per cent of
  respondents), and remains vital in the diagnosis of dry eye disorders

- The FBUT test is the first choice objective diagnostic test (19 per cent of respondents)
- Fluorescein and rose bengal staining remain the prime clinical methods for detecting ocular surface disorders or disease
- The Schirmer test, despite its reported difficulties, is used by over 60 per cent of those surveyed
- Lipid layer and meibomian gland evaluations are, surprisingly, not commonly employed
- The phenol red test by Hamano has significant acceptance in optometry (30 per cent) but almost no acceptance in ophthalmology (5 per cent)
- Lissamine green is increasing in popularity, being reported by 16 per cent of respondents as one of the four preferred tests, and by another 10 per cent in the comment section; osmolarity was mentioned in the comments by 10 per cent as a test of choice if cost, instrumentation, and clinical implementation were not factors
- The respondents of the survey use those tests that can be administered in a clinically efficient manner, although other resources are often available to them
- Laboratory tests, other than osmolarity, are rarely used; tear film evaporation, tear protein analysis, tear ferning, and impression cytology were not mentioned as one of the four preferred choices by any respondent.

Factors, questions and controversies in tear film evaluation

Tear film stability and break-up time

Introduction

Tear film stability, a subject of immense complexity, has been known to be a common denominator among conditions causing ocular irritation since 1973 (Holly, 1973; Pflugfelder et al., 1998). Break-up time (BUT) is the only clinically applicable method of measuring tear film stability. BUT may be defined as the time interval following a blink to the occurrence of gaps or breaks in the tear film.

Tear film stability can be evaluated by both invasive and non-invasive methods. The invasive method requires the use of fluorescein to determine fluorescein break-up time (FBUT), while non-invasive methods utilize observation of the image of a grid or other pattern directed onto the precorneal tear film (Mengher *et al.*, 1985a; Patel *et al.*, 1985; Tonge *et al.*, 1991; Madden *et al.*, 1994).

Lemp *et al.* (1970, 1971) are credited with establishing that the cut-off point for abnormal tear break-up time values was less than 10 s. It is now generally accepted that an FBUT value of less than 10 s is abnormal (Rengstorff, 1974; Norn, 1992). Values of 5–9 s may be considered marginal dry eye and values of 5 s or less are diagnostic of a dry eye disorder (Mackie and Seal, 1981). The usual ranges reported for normal FBUT values vary; Lemp and Hamill (1973) reported 15–34 s, Rengstorff 10–30 s, and Norn (1969) reported an average value of 26 s, but with wide variations from 3–132 s for subjects considered normal. The normal range for the NIBUT is 40–60 s, which is greater than the values found with the FBUT test (Tonge *et al.*, 1991).

Pflugfelder *et al.* (1998) recently recommended that the FBUT test should be used as the 'first test' and the only test to decide if an eye problem is related to the tear film or to another cause. Further, the statement by the National Eye Institute/industry workshop on clinical trials in dry eyes that 'It is recommended that a test of tear stability (BUT) be used as a global criterion of dry eye' substantiates the unique importance and relevance of BUT measurement (Lemp, 1995).

The above study by Pflugfelder *et al.* (1998) noted that 'an unstable tear film is the hallmark of various dry eye states' and that a significantly faster fluorescein break-up time was a common finding with four primary conditions causing ocular irritation: Sjögren's syndrome-related aqueous tear deficiency; non-Sjögren's syndrome-related aqueous tear deficiency; inflammatory meibomian gland disease associated with rosacea; and atrophic meibomian gland disease. They also pointed out that other investigators have reported rapid FBUT in different types of dry eye conditions, including keratoconjunctivitis sicca (Norn, 1969), mucin deficiency (Lemp *et al.*, 1971), meibomian keratoconjunctivitis (McCulley and Sciallis, 1977) and meibomian dysfunction in rosacea (Zengin *et al.*, 1995). Andres *et al.* (1987) found that 86 per cent of patients with FBUT of < 10 s experienced problems with contact lenses, regardless of whether they were soft or rigid, but that only 2 per cent of patients with normal FBUT developed contact lens intolerance. It would therefore appear that the FBUT test should be an essential component of tear film diagnosis.

However, the survey of 68 practitioners revealed that only 19 per cent used the FBUT test as their first choice test, probably due to variable results, as evidenced by the respondents' comments. The NIBUT test was not used as a first choice test by any respondent and was used by only 4 per cent of respondents. There is sufficient new information to require reconsideration of both the FBUT and NIBUT tests and their methodologies.

Fluorescein break-up time (FBUT) – limitations

FBUT, 30 years after its introduction by Norn as 'corneal wetting time', is criticized as inaccurate, unscientific, or not reproducible and is therefore not universally accepted (Mengher *et al.*, 1985b, 1986; Marquardt *et al.*, 1986). Andres *et al.* (1987) noted that a wide range of average FBUT values, from 15 to > 50 s, was found in separate studies. Further, FBUT has been reported to have no clinical value, since it is dependent upon the amount of fluorescein instilled onto the eye (Larke, 1997). The survey of 68 practitioners disclosed that only 19 per cent used the FBUT as their first choice test and only 50 per cent included FBUT as one of their four preferred tests. Thus, approximately half of this group of practitioners does not routinely use FBUT and, despite its 30 years of existence, the clinical use and value of FBUT is controversial.

The usual rationale to explain the FBUT test's lack of reproducibility is its inherent limitation as an invasive technique, thereby altering tear film stability and compromising the test (Mengher *et al.*, 1985b; Marquardt *et al.*, 1986). A critical factor resulting in non-reproducible FBUT measurements is the volume of fluorescein used (Marquardt *et al.*, 1986). (Other variables include the concentration and the pH of the fluorescein solution, the intensity and nature of the illumination and excitation filters, and the time following instillation of the fluorescein to commencement of the test.) Norn (1969) originally chose a low concentration of fluorescein of 0.125 per cent and a drop size of 10 µl (one-fifth the size of a normal drop) to standardize conditions. Norn's emphasis on using a standard volume of fluorescein solution has not usually been implemented because of the time and difficulty in customizing concentrations and volumes. As a result, the test is usually performed with either fluorescein impregnated paper or with a drop of unspecified size of 1 per cent or 2 per cent fluorescein. The literature is frequently not clear as to either the volume or the concentration of fluorescein used in performing FBUT, leading to additional variability and compromising the reproducibility of results.

The fluorescein strip is prepared for application by moistening with one or several drops of balanced, unpreserved saline. While some investigators recommend shaking the strip prior to instillation (Marquardt *et al.*, 1986; Lowther, 1997), others do not make a specific recommendation (Lemp and Hamill, 1973; Nelson, 1994). The strip is then touched to either the superior (Lowther, 1997), inferior (Lemp and Hamill, 1973; Norn, 1992), temporal (Marquardt *et al.*, 1986), or inferior temporal (Pflugfelder *et al.*, 1998) bulbar conjunctiva, or to the tear meniscus (Nelson, 1994). However, the volume of fluorescein delivered to the eye by the fluorescein strip for the FBUT test has not been reported. Snyder and Paugh (1998) recently reported that the volume of fluid delivered by standard rose bengal impregnated strips is 17.43 µl (±3.09) after wetting with 100 µl (two drops) of sterile saline and allowing the excess saline to fall off the strip by gravity. Since the physical dimensions of the rose bengal and fluorescein strips are identical, it would appear that both would deliver similar volumes of fluid. The total volume of the tear film of the eye is only 7 µl, therefore adding over twice the total tear volume to the eye for the evaluation of FBUT will destabilize the tear film and compromise the measurement of tear film stability.

Thus, both the large volume of fluorescein in relation to the total volume of the tear film and the difficulty in standardizing the volume delivered from the strip contribute to the lack of reproducibility. Reflex tearing from physically touching the palpebral conjunctiva and instilling a greater volume of fluorescein than that of the tear film are additional potential sources of variability. The results of the FBUT test with the fluorescein strip are very dependent upon the expertise of the practitioner in controlling the many variables, minimizing the disturbance to the tear film and avoiding reflex tearing.

The use of fluorescein solution also presents problems. When a standard drop of 40–50 µl is applied to the normal volume of 7–10 µl of tear fluid within the palpebral aperture, approximately five times the normal tear volume is added with resulting tear film disruption. Andres *et al.* (1987) used one drop of fluorescein solution and commented that the FBUT values were low (12.8 ± 3.5 s). They suggested that the use of a drop of fluorescein, rather than strips which would have delivered smaller volumes of fluorescein, might have contributed to the low FBUT values. Although Norn's (1969) original proposal considered the volume and concentration of the fluorescein, subsequent investigators and clinicians have generally abandoned specific controls for volume and concentration in favour of simply using commercially available products.

An improved FBUT test would require utilizing the smallest possible controlled volume of fluorescein, thus minimizing the two primary variables, disruption of the tear film and control of volume.

FBUT modifications

Marquardt *et al.* (1986) compared the break-up time findings using fluorescein strips to a technique using 1–2 µl of 5 per cent fluorescein solution applied with a laboratory ultra micro digital pipette. They reported an increase in the reliability with the 1–2 µl solution method. A subsequent investigation has confirmed the improved reproducibility of FBUT findings with Marquardt's technique (Korb *et al.*, 1999). The introduction of the minimal volume of fluorescein required to obtain adequate fluorescence presents the ideal theoretical model for FBUT evaluation. If 1 μl or less of fluorescein could be delivered for the FBUT test by a method suitable for routine clinical use, it would become the method of choice and the gold standard. However, the instillation of micro amounts of fluorescein has required the use of specialized equipment such as laboratory ultra micro digital pipettes and a separate source of liquid fluorescein. This method also appears both invasive and threatening to the patient and could be potentially hazardous in routine clinical use since laboratory pipettes are not designed for ophthalmic use. Other techniques include the use of syringes for control of the volume of fluorescein (Rengstorff, 1974); however, they are also not clinically practical.

Another consideration is the time required after the instillation of the fluorescein for the tear film to stabilize. The length of this waiting period depends upon the volume and concentration instilled, and the fluorescein achieving an appropriate concentration and fluorescence for making the FBUT observation. Following instillation of 1 μl of two per cent fluorescein solution, only 5–15 s are required for the tear film to stabilize so that reproducible FBUT measurements can be made. However, with 15 μl of fluorescein, a longer waiting period of up to 12 minutes may be required for reproducible FBUT findings. Thus, the greater the volume of fluorescein instilled, the longer the time required for the tear film to stabilize, a requirement for reproducible FBUT measurements.

Fluorescein concentration and fluorescence

The phenomenon of fluorescence is concentration-dependent. A common clinical observation is that fluorescein may not fluoresce immediately after initial instillation and may require the addition of saline to achieve fluorescence (Korb and Korb, 1970; Norn, 1970). When fluorescein is used for tear film evaluation, the resulting fluorescence is dependent on both the concentration and the volume which is instilled onto the eye. The concentration of fluorescein that should be used is thought to depend on the volume instilled; the smaller the volume the greater the concentration required. Marquardt et al. (1986) have recommended the use of 5 per cent fluorescein if small volumes of 1–2 μl are used. However, it has also been reported that the higher the concentration of fluorescein, the lower the FBUT value (Vanley et al., 1977).

Finnemore et al. (1998) evaluated the degree of fluorescence obtained after 1 μl volumes of 2 per cent and 10 per cent fluorescein concentrations were instilled onto the inferior palpebral conjunctiva of subjects, aged 20–50, with FBUT times of > 10 s, Schirmer tests of > 10 mm, and lipid layer thicknesses ≥ 90 nm. Two per cent fluorescein solution produced an immediate grade 3 fluorescence (maximum fluorescence on a scale of

0–3); however, the 10 per cent fluorescein solution required an average of 2.2 minutes to achieve the same level of fluorescence. The duration of the maximum fluorescence with 10 per cent fluorescein solution was longer (13.4 ± 4.33 minutes) than that observed with the 2 per cent fluorescein solution (6.35 ± 1.57 minutes). When a given volume and concentration of fluorescein is instilled onto the tear film, it must be diluted by the tears before it will fluoresce. Aqueous-deficient tear films required a longer time for the 10 per cent concentration of fluorescein to be adequately diluted to produce fluorescence. This appears to be the result of self-quenching of fluorescence caused by a high concentration of fluorescein molecules in the upper layers of the tear film (Wilson *et al.*, 1995). Summarizing, this study demonstrated that 1 µl of 10 per cent fluorescein solution requires several minutes to be adequately diluted to produce fluorescence, while 1 µl of 2 per cent fluorescein solution produces immediate and maximum fluorescence.

Clinical procedures

Since tear film stability appears to be a very useful, if not a critical factor in the diagnosis of a broad spectrum of tear disorder conditions, an FBUT test which is repeatable in the hands of the clinician is very desirable. Pflugfelder (1996) referring to the FBUT test reported: 'Although far from ideal, the best clinical test currently available for identifying tear film instability is the fluorescein (or invasive) tear break-up time measurement.' Possible techniques for use in the routine office setting include:

Standard clinical techniques
The clinician may select one of many recommended techniques utilizing commercially available fluorescein strips. The challenge is to obtain a repeatable volume and concentration of fluorescein and to avoid ocular sensation and reflex tearing. The technique of Nelson (1994), which has been recommended by Pflugfelder (1996), touches the strip to the tear meniscus rather than the ocular surface. Although this technique requires significant clinical expertise, it deserves consideration as a method of choice, since it reduces the volume of fluorescein instilled onto the eye. This technique uses 'several' drops of saline for wetting the strip and does not recommend shaking off the excess.

Nelson technique for measuring fluorescein tear break-up time (TBUT)
- Apply several drops of unpreserved solution to a fluorescein strip
- Gently touch the strip to the inferior tear meniscus
- Ask the patient to blink and roll the eyes around several times
- Wait 1 minute

- Ask the patient to close the eyes and then keep them open
- Measure (in seconds) the time between eye opening and appearance of the first dry spot
- Record the mean of three trials.

Lowther technique for measuring fluorescein tear break-up time

A slightly different technique, which advocates shaking off the excessive fluorescein, has been recommended by Lowther (1997).

- Moisten a fluorescein strip with buffered, non-preserved saline
- Shake excess solution off
- Gently touch the strip to the superior bulbar conjunctiva or lid margin, taking care not to instil too much solution or cause excessive reflex tearing
- Instruct the patient to blink two or three times
- Keep the eyes open naturally – do not exaggerate the opening.

The advantages of these techniques are the ease of application, clinical applicability, and immediacy of results. The disadvantages are lack of control over volume and/or concentration of the instilled fluorescein, and possible sensation resulting in reflex tearing.

A new modification of the FBUT test, the DET test

The report of Marquardt *et al.* (1986) that a volume of 1 µl of 2 per cent fluorescein solution instilled into the tear film provides a more accurate and repeatable method of quantifying tear film break-up time has been recently confirmed (Korb *et al.*, 1999). If the volume is increased over 1 µl, the findings become less reliable.

Recognizing the need for a clinically applicable FBUT test that would provide results comparable to the ultra micro digital pipette method with 1–2 µl of 2 per cent fluorescein, but without the disadvantages and patient apprehension, Korb *et al.* (1999) have developed a new fluorescein strip test. The goals of this new strip are to:

1. Duplicate the delivery of 1 µl of 2 per cent fluorescein solution to the tear film by the pipette method
2. Accomplish the instillation of the fluorescein without sensation
3. Avoid disruption of the tear film
4. Eliminate the need to shake the strip and the resulting inherent variability of the delivered volume
5. Eliminate the waiting period after instillation of the fluorescein prior to the FBUT measurement.

The standard fluorescein impregnated strip is approximately 5 mm wide by 15 mm long and 75 mm^2 (Abdul-Fattah *et al.*, 1999), and delivers approximately 17 μl of fluid to the eye after wetting (Snyder and Paugh, 1998). A surface area of 7.5 mm^2 of fluorescein impregnated strip, after wetting with sterile saline, will deliver the same amount of fluorescein (0.020 mg) to the tear film when touched to the bulbar conjunctiva for 1–2 seconds as 1 μl of 2 per cent fluorescein solution (Abdul-Fattah *et al.*, 1999; Korb *et al.*, 1999). If the configuration of the new strip is ≤1.0 mm wide, shaking is not necessary since, after wetting with sterile saline, the excess fluid will fall from the strip, providing the desired delivery of a 1 μl volume of fluorescein solution to the ocular surface. It was found that the ideal dimensions for the fluorescein impregnated strip are 1.0 mm wide by 7.5 mm long. This provides a design which, when applied to the bulbar conjunctiva, delivers the desired volume of 1 μl containing the 0.020 mg of fluorescein required for fluorescence, allowing the test to be used with greater ease than a standard strip and without sensation.

The characteristics of the fluorescence of the tear film provided by the new strip technique were compared by several methods to that provided by 1 μl of 2 per cent fluorescein solution delivered by the ultra micro digital pipette, and were found to be the same for both techniques (Abdul-Fattah *et al.*, 1999). Adequate fluorescence for FBUT observation was achieved immediately after instillation of the fluorescein with both methods. The duration of the fluorescence for a given eye was the same for both methods, varying from 1.5–5.0 minutes as a function of the tear turnover rate. Thus, the new technique duplicates the 1 μl volume delivered by the pipette without its disadvantages. This new strip is marketed as the DET test by Akorn Inc., Buffalo Grove, Illinois. (The author has an ownership interest in Ocular Research of Boston, a company commercializing dry eye products and the developer of the DET test.)

Method for measuring FBUT with the DET test to deliver 1 μl of fluorescein solution

- Apply one or two drops of non-preserved saline to the impregnated fluorescein paper tip; excess fluid will automatically fall off and shaking of the strip is neither required nor desirable
- Ask the patient to look down and in
- Gently touch the strip to the superior temporal bulbar conjunctiva for 1–2 s
- Ask the patient to blink three times and open the eyes naturally
- Conduct the FBUT measurement immediately
- Perform two consecutive measurements; if not consistent, conduct a third measurement and average
- Repeat for the second eye.

The 'soak time', as pointed out by Snyder and Paugh (1998), influences the concentration of dye (rose bengal) delivered to the eye with impregnated strips. They found a 34 per cent increase in concentration if the soak time was increased from 15 s to 45 s. Our studies investigated this variable and found that it was not a significant factor with the new strip in providing the fluorescence required for the FBUT test. It is therefore not necessary to control soak time with this method.

This new technique provides a simplified method of delivery of consistent volumes of fluorescein solution of 1 μl with more accurate and repeatable FBUT measurements.

Non-invasive break-up time (NIBUT)

NIBUT measurement utilizes a grid or other pattern directed onto the precorneal tear film for the observation of distortion and/or abnormality in the image. The time interval in seconds following a blink to the first change of the image is defined as the NIBUT. This method eliminates physical disturbance to the tear film from the instillation of fluorescein, along with the possibility of inducing reflex tearing. Measuring NIBUT would therefore appear to be both an ideal theoretical and a more realistic method of evaluating tear film stability than FBUT and would be expected to provide more reliable and reproducible results.

The values for BUT found with the NIBUT test are significantly greater than the values found with the FBUT test. The normal range for NIBUT is 40–60 s (Tonge et al., 1991) as compared to normal ranges of 10–34 s (Lemp and Hamill, 1973; Rengstorff, 1974) for the FBUT. The longer NIBUT values were first reported by Marx in 1921 and then by Go Ing Hovn in 1926, who observed (without a slit lamp or fluorescein) that dry spots occurred in the tear film after 60–67 s, but with substantial variability (Murube, 1992). While the first instrument for the evaluation of NIBUT was reported by Mengher et al. (1985a), an instrument solely dedicated to NIBUT measurement has never been made commercially available. The Tearscope Plus™ (Keeler Instruments, Broomall, PA) may be used for NIBUT by utilizing accessory removable grids (Tearscope Plus, 1997). Currently, as might be expected, the use of the NIBUT test in clinical practice is minimal. The NIBUT test (using either custom instruments or the Tearscope Plus™ with accessory grids) was reported by only 5 per cent of respondents in the survey as part of their diagnostic procedure.

A new role for the NIBUT technique, assessing the integrity and stability of the precorneal mucin layer, was presented by Pflugfelder et al. (1998). Utilizing the xeroscope, a prototype instrument, to measure NIBUT, they reported that NIBUT was a useful measurement for differentiating aqueous tear deficiency (ATD) from meibomian gland disease (MGD). The authors reported grid distortions were present immediately after a blink in a significantly greater percentage of subjects with ATD, particularly the Sjögren's syndrome group, than in a meibomian gland disease group. They reported that none of the eyes in the meibomian gland disease group showed this type of grid abnormality. A positive correlation was found between the NIBUT grid distortions and the mean Schirmer test scores.

The authors also hypothesized that NIBUT evaluated a different phenomenon than FBUT and that the distortions noted by NIBUT might be the result of a deficiency in the tear mucous layer. The rationale for their hypothesis was based on a strong positive correlation between the NIBUT grid distortions and rose bengal staining, since corneal rose bengal staining is thought to result from a deficiency of the precorneal mucous layer. The precorneal mucous layer was removed and a similar grid appearance to those seen in patients with ATD was observed, confirming the hypothesis that the NIBUT grid distortions appearing immediately after the blink were due to a deficiency in the tear mucous layer. Referring to NIBUT, they reported that the xeroscope could be used as a valuable non-invasive technique for assessing integrity and stability of the precorneal mucin layer. This proposal of a specific use for NIBUT for the diagnosis of tear mucous layer deficiency may provide impetus for further development of NIBUT instrumentation and increased use of this technique.

This study concluded that NIBUT was valuable for the diagnosis of tear film mucous layer deficiencies, but that it did not replace the FBUT test as the first choice test for the evaluation of tear film stability

Summary of break-up time

- Fluorescein break-up time (FBUT), although not ideal, is the best clinical test currently available for identifying tear film instability
- The primary problem with the FBUT test has been that the measurements are not reproducible. The smaller the volume of fluorescein used, the more reproducible the FBUT measurement. Several clinical suggestions and techniques to improve this problem are offered. A new FBUT test by Korb *et al.* (1999), known as the DET test, instils 1 µl of fluorescein solution onto the ocular surface. This technique will produce identical results to those achieved with 1 µl of fluorescein solution delivered by ultra micro digital pipette
- FBUT values of < 10 s are considered abnormal, values of 5–9 s are borderline dry eye, and values of < 5 s are clearly indicative of dry eye disorder

- The first choice objective test of clinicians for diagnosis of the tear film and dry eye is the FBUT test
- A concentration of 2 per cent fluorescein is adequate for the FBUT test, even for micro volumes of 1 µl
- Non-invasive break-up time (NIBUT) presents an ideal theoretical method to measure tear film stability; however, it is not in routine clinical use since instrumentation is not commercially available. NIBUT values are two to four times greater than those found with FBUT; the rationale for this difference has not been completely explained. Pflugfelder *et al.* (1998) reported that the NIBUT test is useful since it evaluates a different phenomenon than the FBUT test (the integrity of the precorneal mucin layer), but does not replace the FBUT test as the first choice test for tear film stability
- Although the NIBUT test does not replace the FBUT test, it nevertheless has a role in tear film diagnosis.

Ocular surface staining

Introduction

Since damage to the ocular surface is a result of dry eye disorders, evaluating the ocular surface is an important part of the diagnosis of the dry eye. A number of techniques are available for this purpose, including impression cytology (Adams, 1979; Nelson, 1982; Egbert *et al.*, 1997), microscopy with sloughed cells (Norn, 1960; Lohman *et al.*, 1982; Fullard and Wilson, 1986) and specular microscopy (Lohman *et al.*, 1982; Lemp and Mathers, 1986). However, ocular surface staining provides the most convenient and clinically feasible approach.

Why are stains used?

Damage to the ocular surface is recognized as one of the three factors necessary for a disorder to be included within the 'global definition' of dry eye disorders by the National Eye Institute/industry workshop on clinical trials in dry eyes (Lemp, 1995). The result of dry eye disorders, including those in which the tear film is not adequately protecting the corneal and conjunctival epithelium, is a damaged, altered, or compromised epithelium and/or its associated tight junctions. The use of stains allows the direct, and usually immediate, observation of these abnormalities.

The clinical importance of staining is reflected in the survey results, which revealed that the majority of respondents (>75 per cent) use one or more dyes to appraise ocular surface features as part of their tear film/

dry eye evaluation. Twenty-five per cent of respondents used fluorescein or rose bengal as their first choice test for dry eye evaluation. Rose bengal was used as one of four preferred tests by 50 per cent of respondents, fluorescein by 48 per cent and lissamine green by 15 per cent.

Questions and controversies

Given the prominent role of ocular surface staining in the diagnostic evaluation of dry eye, it is appropriate to review the three commonly used stains (fluorescein, rose bengal and lissamine green), staining procedures and their interpretation, particularly in light of current research which raises interesting questions and issues that may challenge long-held concepts. The questions and controversies include:

- Do the stains have a specific action?
- Do normal healthy cells stain?
- Are the cells that are stained live or dead?
- Are these stains toxic?
- Is there an optimal stain concentration and volume?
- What is the duration of time between instillation and observation?
- Is sequential staining indicated?
- What are the frequency and implications of corneal staining with apparently normal healthy eyes?
- How is staining graded?
- How are the findings interpreted?

These are clinically relevant questions and the goals of this section are to summarize current knowledge in this area and provide recommendations for the clinician to use in daily practice.

Specific actions and interpretations

Fluorescein

Fluorescein has been used on the human cornea for over 100 years (Straub, 1888, cited in Norn, 1974). It has been generally accepted, based on the fundamental observations of Norn (1970), that fluorescein only penetrates into the corneal epithelium at the sites of interrupted continuity of the epithelial surface and discloses lesions of the corneal epithelium. Norn's findings have remained unchallenged since their publication three decades ago. Feenstra and Tseng (1992a) support Norn's concept that fluorescein, when viewed under blue-light and the biomicro-scope, does not stain healthy, dead, or degenerated cells, and that the staining is essentially limited to the disruption of the cell–cell junctions and subsequent diffusion of fluorescein. However, they also found that cultured rabbit corneal epithelial cells demonstrated fluorescein staining when viewed with a fluorescence microscope.

Wilson *et al.* (1995) detected that individual corneal cells would stain with fluorescein and that the staining of these individual cells could be observed with the biomicroscope and 16X magnification. Intensely fluorescent cells were interpreted as being those that had taken up fluorescein at the optimum concentration for fluorescence. These authors reported that fainter staining and the typical 'salt and pepper' (darkened) appearance resulted from a quenching phenomenon where the intensity of fluorescence declined for those cells that had taken up a greater than optimum concentration of fluorescein. There was no indication in this study that fluorescein staining was due to the filling of intercellular spaces or areas of cell drop-out. Whether fluorescein stains healthy, compromised or dead epithelial cells, or cell–cell junctions, or all of these, it still remains the mainstay in the detection of defects of the corneal surface.

Fluorescein staining, even if micropunctate, is considered to be a danger signal for dry eye disorders (Norn, 1970). Significant fluorescein staining of the cornea has also been correlated with contact lens intolerance (Korb and Herman, 1979). Fluorescein staining appears to offer the best clinical method of diagnosing the presence of epithelial surface defects, particularly for those conditions of lesser severity than would be stained by rose bengal. These conditions include the 'marginal dry eye' and moderate dry eye states. Thus, fluorescein staining of the cornea is particularly valuable for the detection of surface defects with marginal to moderate dry eye disorders.

Fluorescein staining of the cornea is usually associated with dry eye disorders or corneal exposure problems. However, as pointed out by Mackie and Seal (1981), both fluorescein and rose bengal corneal staining may occur with staphylococcal disease, ocular rosacea, allergic disease and other disease entities. These possibilities should be considered in the diagnosis.

In summary, fluorescein staining is the premier method for the diagnosis of epithelial defects, although there is controversy as to the exact structures which are stained.

Rose bengal

Rose bengal was first used on the eye in 1914 (Römer *et al.*, cited in Norn, 1974) and was popularized by Sjögren in 1933 (Norn, 1974) for the diagnosis of keratoconjunctivitis sicca. It has been generally agreed, based upon Norn's (1972) early work, that rose bengal stains dead or degenerated epithelial cells and mucus, including the mucous thread.

In contrast, Feenstra and Tseng (1992b) have demonstrated that rose bengal stains healthy cultured rabbit corneal epithelial cells. This staining, which was visible without the aid of a microscope, could be blocked by coating the cultured cells with solutions of mucin or albumin prior to the staining procedure. This result has led to the speculation that the apparent inability of rose bengal to stain corneal epithelial cells *in vivo* is a reflection of the presence of analogous blocking factors in the tear film or in the mucin layer immediately overlying these cells. In fact, treatment of normal rabbit corneal epithelium with acetylcysteine, a mucolytic agent, enhances rose bengal staining, lending further support to the theory that the staining ability of rose bengal *in vivo* is a function of the 'blocking status' of the precorneal tear film.

Thus, by extrapolation, the presence of rose bengal staining of the cornea *in vivo* may be interpreted as an indication of a deficiency of preocular tear film protection. Whether the cells stained by rose bengal are healthy, compromised or dead requires further clarification.

Rose bengal staining is more commonly found on the exposed conjunctival epithelium than on the cornea. Rose bengal staining of the exposed bulbar conjunctival epithelium frequently occurs with adults, particularly nasally and on raised areas. Unless the staining is moderate or severe, it is accepted as normal. Norn (1974) has reported that rose bengal staining on the bulbar conjunctiva, most often inferiorly and nasally, is normal for elderly eyes.

Rose bengal is the ideal dye for evaluating the protective status of the preocular tear film (Tseng, 1994), the result of its staining epithelial cells which are not protected by a healthy tear mucous layer. Rose bengal also stains dead and degenerated cells and maintains its premier position for the diagnosis of keratoconjunctivitis sicca (KCS). In the early stages of KCS the conjunctiva stains. As the disease progresses the cornea then stains, and in severe KCS the entire cornea may stain (Nelson, 1994). Rose bengal staining occurring with moderate or severe aqueous tear deficiency, as found with KCS, is typically confined to the interpalpebral (open eye) exposed zone of the cornea and conjunctiva.

While the staining of the cornea by rose bengal appears to be a function of the degree of mucus protection (Feenstra and Tseng, 1992b), the staining of the conjunctiva by rose bengal does not appear to have as ready an explanation. Although mild rose bengal staining of the conjunctiva is common, rose bengal staining of the cornea is relatively uncommon and usually limited to pathological conditions. Determining the clinical relevance of rose bengal staining of the conjunctiva and cornea requires consideration of whether this staining is a normal finding for the given individual or signifies inadequate mucous layer protection for healthy cells, the staining of devitalized or dead cells, or possibly both. The answer is dependent on the particular patient profile and the results of other diagnostic tests.

Surprisingly, corneal mechanical abrasions stain minimally or not at all with rose bengal, but stain acutely with fluorescein. With KCS there is minimal to moderate staining with fluorescein, but severe staining with rose bengal. Corneal infiltrates infrequently stain with rose bengal but may stain with fluorescein, which is considered an important diagnostic criterion for treatment and for contact lens management.

Bron (1997) presented a generally accepted view when he pointed out: 'The standard method to demonstrate ocular surface damage is to stain the ocular surface with fluorescein to show corneal damage and with bengal rose to show damage on the bulbar conjunctiva.'

Lissamine green

Lissamine green was introduced by Norn (1973) as having identical properties to rose bengal. It is considered non-toxic and does not sting and therefore has been suggested as a replacement for rose bengal. Lissamine green has been reported by Tseng (1994) to be ideal for the detection of dead or degenerate cells and will not stain healthy cells. However, this stain does not appear to be a substitute for rose bengal, since it will not provide an evaluation of the protective status of the mucous layer.

The use of stains is summarized in Table 6.4.

Although there is controversy as to the specific mechanisms of action and possible interpretation of staining, the important aspect is that each of the three stains behaves very differently on the ocular surface. Fluorescein and rose bengal have a long history of productive use in the diagnosis of tear film and ocular surface conditions. The clinician who is comfortable with the use of these stains for their diagnostic potential should maintain their habitual use and clinical interpretation, while considering how to incorporate the new information to further enhance his/her clinical routine.

Summary of specific actions

- Fluorescein is the dye of choice for demonstrating corneal damage; rose bengal is the preferred dye for staining areas of damage on the bulbar conjunctiva (Bron, 1997)
- Lissamine green is a potential substitute for rose bengal without sting, but does not replace rose bengal's probable ability to diagnose deficiency of the mucous layer.

Are ocular stains toxic?

It has been generally accepted that ocular surface stains are not cytotoxic. In a discussion of the issue of toxicity, it is interesting to include the

Table 6.4 Differences in staining characteristics of ocular dyes (modified from Tseng, 1994)

	Fluorescein	*Rose bengal*	*Lissamine green B*
Stains cells	Uncertain and complex*	Yes	Yes
Stains healthy cells		Yes, if unprotected by mucus (Feenstra and Tseng, 1992)	No
Stains compromised cells	Yes (Wilson *et al.*, 1995)	Yes	Yes
Site of staining	Disruptions of cell–cell junctions (Norn, 1970; Feenstra and Tseng, 1992) and/or cell damage (Wilson *et al.*, 1995)	Stains cell nuclei	Similar to rose bengal
Relative speed for stromal diffusion	Very fast	Slow (Feenstra and Tseng, 1992)	Fast
Staining blocked by mucin	No	Yes (Feenstra and Tseng, 1992)	No
Intrinsic toxicity	No	Yes (Feenstra and Tseng, 1992)	No data
Phototoxicity	No	Yes (Feenstra and Tseng, 1992)	No data
Sting potential	No	Yes – varies from mild to very severe	No
Clinical implications	The optimal clinical method to demonstrate corneal damage (Bron, 1997)	Standard method to demonstrate damage on the bulbar conjunctiva (Bron, 1997); refer to text for other indications	Potential substitute for rose bengal without sting, but cannot diagnose deficiency of the mucous layer

*Fluorescein stains healthy cells poorly and is detected only by the laboratory microscope (Feenstra and Tseng, 1992; Tseng, 1994). Fluorescein stains individual cells, including those not most physiologically compromised. Fluorescein staining may be seen with clinical biomicroscope (Wilson *et al.*, 1995).

observation of Paracelsus (1493–1541) who noted that: 'All substances are poisons; there is none which is not a poison. The right dose differentiates a poison and a remedy' (Klaassen, 1980). Klaassen expanded on this idea by pointing out that the primary concern in toxicology is the risk or hazard associated with the use of a chemical, not whether the chemical itself is safe or toxic. In fact, it has been reported that 0.9 per cent sodium chloride (i.e. normal saline) alone induces toxic effects on conjunctival epithelium in culture, beginning 3–5 minutes after initial exposure (Merrill *et al.*, 1960). It is within this framework that the question of stain toxicity should be approached.

There is a high probability that rose bengal is toxic to epithelial cells as demonstrated by its cytotoxicity *in vitro* (Feenstra and Tseng, 1992b). Additionally, rose bengal has been reported to have a phototoxic effect on cultured cells (Feenstra and Tseng, 1992b). Clinical use of rose bengal may result in stinging, from mild to very severe, offering support for its toxicity. There is no evidence that lissamine green is toxic to corneal or conjunctival epithelium. Fluorescein has been used on the human cornea for over 100 years (Norn, 1974) and is considered non-toxic (Tseng, 1994); however, Thomas *et al.* (1997) have reported that sodium fluorescein is cytotoxic to human corneal epithelial cells, particularly under conditions of sequential staining. This is in contrast to other reports that failed to demonstrate an intrinsic toxicity with sodium fluorescein *in vitro* (Feenstra and Tseng, 1992a; Tseng, 1994). Differences in experimental *in vivo* and *in vitro* models, concentrations of fluorescein used, and liquid *vs.* impregnated strip methods of application may explain, in part, the discrepancies between these studies. It should be noted that sodium fluorescein solution in 10 per cent concentration is routinely used intravenously to study retinal and choroidal circulation. This is a significantly higher concentration than the 1–2 per cent solutions routinely used to stain the ocular surface and offers support for fluorescein being considered non-toxic.

In summary, fluorescein and lissamine green may be considered non-toxic, while rose bengal appears somewhat toxic when used topically on the eye. Nevertheless, the ocular side-effects due to these ophthalmic dyes should be considered rare and transient (Fraunfelder, 1996).

Is there an optimal concentration and volume of dye for clinical staining?

It has been shown that staining is concentration dependent for both fluorescein and rose bengal (Norn, 1974; Feenstra and Tseng, 1992a; Tseng 1994). It is therefore essential to use an adequate volume and concentration of dye to obtain consistent and useful results. Dyes are available in strip and liquid forms. Using liquid drops is the only method that guarantees a constant concentration of dye (Norn, 1974; Tseng 1994). If fluorescein impregnated strips are used to detect staining, the volume and concentration delivered will vary and, if the amount of fluorescein is inadequate, staining may not be visible.

The conflicting opinions as to the optimal volume and concentration of fluorescein and rose bengal for ocular surface staining are based on several factors. If the amount of dye is not adequate, staining will not be observed, suggesting the use of drops of adequate concentration. No contraindications to a conventional drop size of 40–50 µl have been reported for fluorescein. Stinging, varying from marginally perceptible to disabling pain, has been reported for rose bengal, resulting in the recommendation of smaller volumes to minimize stinging (Nelson, 1994).

In two studies of corneal staining with normal populations, Norn (1970) used 10 µl of 0.125 per cent fluorescein solution, while Korb and Korb (1970) used a standard 40–50 µl drop of 2 per cent fluorescein solution. Norn's recommendation for 10 µl was based on the recognition that the approximate volume that the eye could hold was 10 µl. Since Norn's (1992) original publication, he changed his recommendation to 10 µl of 1 per cent fluorescein solution. The majority of reports do not specify either the volume of fluorescein solution or the concentration used in the respective studies. Most studies of fluorescein corneal staining, however, have used impregnated fluorescein strips (Caffery and Josephson, 1991; Bron, 1997; Thomas et al., 1997), resulting in less than optimal control of concentration and volume. Other investigators have recommended the use of drops for fluorescein staining (Korb, 1979; Josephson and Caffery, 1992; Tseng, 1994).

Nelson (1994) advocates using only 5 µl of rose bengal to minimize stinging. Pflugfelder et al. (1998) recommend 20 µl of 1 per cent rose bengal. Norn (1992) reported that the quantity of rose bengal utilized for staining was a 'moot point', with volumes of 2.5 µl to a full drop of 1 per cent rose bengal used.

Summary of concentration and volume of dye
- Liquid dyes are recommended for optimal observation of surface epithelial staining; techniques utilizing impregnated strips may not be adequate
- The concentration of fluorescein should be 2 per cent and the volume 10 µl or greater (standard size drops are not contraindicated, and are probably preferable to ensure adequate fluorescein to detect marginal staining)
- The concentration of rose bengal should be 1 per cent; the volume does not appear to be as critical as with fluorescein, and 5 µl and

greater volumes appear to produce consistent results. Standard drop sizes may be used; however, the concern is excessive stinging on compromised eyes

- Data are not available for the volume of lissamine green, but it would appear that a volume of 10 μl or greater is acceptable.

What is the optimal time interval between dye instillation and observation?

There are no established standards for the waiting period following instillation of the dye prior to observation. Most reports of corneal staining do not state a recommended waiting period. For fluorescein staining, Norn (1992) recommends repeated examinations within the first few minutes to distinguish between genuine and false staining. Norn's (1970) original recommendation was to have the patient blink several times prior to observing, and then repeat the observation after 1–2 minutes to detect the finest staining. Korb and Korb's (1970) study utilized six complete blinks and a minimum wait of 60 s. Pflugfelder *et al.* (1998) recommend waiting several minutes. Irrigation is not required to assess the staining providing the observation is made after 1–2 minutes, since the concentration of fluorescein in the tear film is sufficiently diluted so that it does not obscure observation. If irrigation is used, a wait of 1–2 minutes should be retained prior to the irrigation to guarantee penetration of the stain.

For rose bengal staining, Norn (1992) recommends waiting 1–2 minutes after instillation, prior to observation, for the excess dye on the precorneal film to disappear. Pflugfelder *et al.* (1998) recommend a wait of 2 minutes. Tseng (1994) recommends that rose bengal be irrigated immediately after instillation due to the dye's intrinsic toxicity and photosensitizing toxic effects, and that interpretation also be performed immediately.

Summary of time between dye instillation and observation
- A recommended clinical procedure for either fluorescein or rose bengal staining is to instil the dye, blink three times, wait 1–2 minutes to guarantee penetration into the epithelium, and observe
- Staining may be masked immediately after the initial instillation by excess dye in the tear film. Waiting 1–2 minutes will allow the dye in the tear film to dilute so that observation is not obscured. Irrigation is not required; if irrigation is used, the waiting period prior to irrigation should still be retained to allow adequate penetration into the epithelium.

Is sequential staining indicated?

Sequential staining with fluorescein was introduced by Korb and Herman (1979). It was found that as a result of the sequential staining process, an additional 20 per cent of corneas exhibited staining. The authors concluded that additional fluorescein instillations over time increased both the prevalence and the severity of epithelial staining. Caffery and Josephson (1991) studied sequential staining in subjects over the course of 30 days and found both significant staining and variability. In a second study, Josephson and Caffery (1992), found a remarkably high percentage of non-contact lens wearers with corneal staining following sequential staining with fluorescein.

Sequential staining, as determined by the survey of 68 practitioners, is not routinely utilized but its advocates find that it will reveal staining of significance when usual fluorescein staining will not. The study of sequential staining by Korb and Herman (1979) found that only 1 per cent of 200 corneas exhibited grade 2 or greater staining with one instillation of 2 per cent fluorescein, but 14 per cent exhibited grade 2 or 3 staining after sequential instillations. Significant staining of grade 2 or 3, as determined by sequential staining, was eight times more prevalent with the group unable to tolerate contact lenses than with groups without contact lens wearing experience or with successful wearing experience.

Clinically, sequential staining may be performed along with other routine ocular examination procedures so that it does not consume excessive time. The author recommends three instillations of 2 per cent fluorescein solution by drops at 3–5 minute intervals to minimize total time. Fluorescein sequential staining is the author's preferred test to disclose mild to moderate corneal surface compromise.

There are no published reports of either rose bengal or lissamine green sequential staining.

Grading staining and comments on observation

The grading of staining is important for standardization and monitoring (Larke, 1985). The original scale by van Bijsterveld (1969) was designed for rose bengal and the evaluation of KCS. Scoring was provided for three areas, the medial and lateral bulbar conjunctiva and the cornea, each section on a scale from 1–3 points, with a maximum score of 9. This scale is still important for the grading of KCS. A further addition to this scale would be the recording of conjunctival staining relative to the exposed or non-exposed zones of the bulbar conjunctiva, since the staining patterns characteristic of aqueous-deficient dry eyes should involve the exposure zone more than the non-exposure zone.

It was found that the original scale developed by van Bijsterveld for rose bengal staining was not ideal for fluorescein staining. When the severity and location of fluorescein staining on the cornea became a subject of significant interest, other scales were developed (Brown *et al.*, 1989; Lemp, 1995). Recently two new scales have been published, the CCLRU (Cornea and Contact Lens Research Unit, University of New South Wales) grading scale and the Efron contact lens grading scale (CCLRU, 1997; Efron, 1998). The Efron scale provides a convenient clinical grading method for contact lens complications; however, the grading for epithelial staining is limited to four grades from mild to severe without consideration of the corneal area, extent, depth, or the presence of conjunctival staining. The CCLRU grading scales are a more complex and comprehensive system that divides the cornea into five areas and then allows the description of the type, extent, and depth of the staining in each area on a scale of 1–4. The CCLRU grading scale is useful for more detailed evaluations, including research purposes. The use of an appropriate scale is critical to establish a baseline and to monitor the progress of any ocular surface problem.

Fluorescence (of fluorescein) may be significantly enhanced on the cornea and conjunctiva, not only by the use of the usual blue filter of the biomicroscope but also by adding a yellow filter (Kodak Wratten 12) over the objective lenses. The highest intensity of illumination possible with the slit lamp using the blue filter will also aid the observation. Rose bengal may be observed in white or red-free light. Lissamine green is best seen with white light.

Corneal staining with apparently normal eyes – prevalence and implications

Fluorescein staining of the cornea with apparently normal eyes (defined as those eyes without ocular or anterior segment pathology or significant reported symptoms) has been reported to occur with a surprisingly high prevalence, the minimum found in any study was 16 per cent (Korb and Korb, 1970; Norn, 1970; Korb and Herman, 1979; Josephson and Caffery, 1992; Thomas *et al.*, 1997). The majority of the staining was grade 1, usually defined as micropunctate (Norn, 1970; CCLRU, 1997), mild and probably within physiological limits (Korb and Herman, 1979), which is also commonly described as minimal superficial staining or stippling. Norn (1970) found that the number of corneas with micropunctate fluorescein staining increased from 4 per cent of normals under 40 years of age to 20 per cent over 50 years of age. (Norn used a weak concentration of 0.125 per cent and 10 µl. A 2 per cent concentration would probably have increased the prevalence of staining.) Following a single instillation of a standard drop of 2 per cent liquid fluorescein, Korb and Herman (1979) found staining above grade 1 in only 1 per cent of 200 corneas; however, following sequential fluorescein staining, 14 per cent of the 200 corneas exhibited grade 2 or grade 3 staining.

As pointed out by Norn (1970), it is difficult to distinguish between physiological fluorescein staining with normal eyes and definite patho-logical fluorescein staining, as the point of transition from one to the other is indefinite. Very slight grade 1 fluorescein staining in human corneas could be interpreted as the result of normal cell desquamation, as reported by Norn (1960) and Fullard and Wilson (1986). Kikkawa (1972) has also reported this phenomenon for rabbits. More severe staining appears to result from other causes.

Corneal fluorescein staining with apparently normal eyes can be a useful diagnostic finding and may suggest that further evaluation and possible treatment is required. If staining is present when other diagnostic findings are negative, a relevant history should be repeated to ascertain whether symptoms are indeed present. Possible causes for staining include meibomian gland dysfunction, partial or impeded blinking, evaporative causes, environment, and ageing. Corneal fluor-escein staining of grade 2 or above, either with a single application of fluorescein or following sequential staining, is usually indicative of a significant tear film disorder and is also an excellent predictor of contact lens intolerance.

Summary

Fluorescein staining

- Fluorescein staining is the premier method for the diagnosis of corneal epithelial defects, although there is controversy as to the exact structures that are stained
- Staining is concentration-dependent for both fluorescein and rose bengal
- Optimal fluorescein staining is achieved with a 2 per cent concentra-tion and instilling a 10 μl or greater volume. Techniques utilizing impregnated strips may not be adequate to obtain sufficient concentration or volume for optimal staining. The recommended procedure is to instil the fluorescein, have the patient blink three times, wait 1–2 minutes and observe. Irrigation is not necessary
- There is no contraindication to the use of standard drop sizes of fluorescein from unit-dose or preserved containers. (This is in direct contrast to the use of fluorescein in BUT testing, where small volumes, preferably micro volumes of 1 μl, are desirable.)
- A contemporary grading scale should be used

- Sequential instillation of fluorescein can reveal significant epithelial staining and surface defects that would otherwise escape detection
- Minimal fluorescein staining (≤ grade 1) has been reported to occur in a surprisingly high percentage of the normal population, indicating a physiological basis for minimal staining
- Grade 3 or 4 fluorescein staining is indicative of a probable dry eye disorder.

Rose bengal staining

- Rose bengal stains dead and degenerated cells and maintains its premier status for the diagnosis of KCS.
- Rose bengal is currently thought to stain epithelium if it is not adequately protected by an intact tear mucous layer.
- Rose bengal should be used at 1 per cent concentration and 5 µl or more for staining. If standard drop sizes (35–50 µl) are used, there is an increased probability of excessive stinging on compromised eyes. Limiting the dose to 5 µl is helpful in controlling stinging. Irrigation following instillation may also be helpful in minimizing stinging.
- Rose bengal staining confined to the interpalpebral (open eye) exposed zone of the cornea and the conjunctiva is usually associated with moderate or severe aqueous deficiency as found with KCS.

Lissamine green staining

- Lissamine green is thought to stain only dead or degenerated cells. It does not appear to be a complete replacement for rose bengal, since it will not provide an evaluation of the protective status of the mucous layer.

The lipid layer

Introduction

The lipid layer is recognized as a critical component of tear film stability and ocular comfort (Korb and Greiner, 1994; Yokoi *et al.*, 1996; Craig and Tomlinson, 1997; Guillon *et al.*, 1997). However, lipid layer evaluation is not routinely employed for diagnosis of dry eye disorders, probably because instrumentation has not been commercially available until recently. Lipid layer thickness (LLT) can be evaluated by the observation of interference phenomena. The high level of contemporary interest in the lipid layer is in great part the result of the work of Jean-Pierre Guillon. His PhD thesis, publications (along with those of Michel Guillon), development of the Tearscope™ (1986) and, more recently, the Tearscope Plus™ have been key stimuli for the recognition of the importance of the lipid layer.

The relevant questions for the clinician are: What tests are required for lipid layer evaluation? How are they performed? How are they graded? And what is their clinical application? This section will address these questions and provide an overview of related considerations.

Characteristics of the lipid layer as determined by interference patterns

Lipid layer thickness (LLT)

The lipid layer may be evaluated by a number of slit-lamp techniques utilizing diffusing filters or additional light sources to create interference phenomena (Ehlers, 1965; McDonald, 1968; Norn, 1979), but the area observed is restricted to several mm^2. These techniques are of limited clinical value because the lipid layer is not uniform in thickness, thus requiring observation of a larger area to reveal the dominant colours and lipid patterns necessary for classification of lipid layer characteristics and LLT. While custom-designed instruments have been developed (Hamano et al., 1982; Josephson, 1983; Guillon, 1987; Korb et al., 1994), at the present time the only commercially available instrument to evaluate the lipid layer is the Tearscope Plus™, designed by Jean-Pierre Guillon and available from Keeler Instruments with a clinical handbook, CD-Rom and instructions. The Tearscope Plus™ projects a cylindrical source of cool white fluorescent light onto the lipid layer illuminating almost all of the corneal surface area. The interference patterns are observed with the magnification of the slit-lamp microscope.

Thicker lipid layers (≥ 90 nm) are readily observed since they result in colour and wave patterns. Thinner lipid layers (≤ 60 nm) are difficult to observe, since colours and distinct morphological features are not present. If the lipid layer is ≤ 50 nm, only a grey or white surface, without other features, is observed (Guillon, 1982; Korb et al., 1994; Tearscope Plus™, 1997). If grey or white waves or flow patterns without colours are seen, the lipid layer is in the range of 50–80 nm.

Guillon (Guillon and Guillon, 1993; Tearscope Plus™, 1997) has proposed five main categories of lipid interference patterns. In order of increasing thickness and visibility they are: open meshwork, closed meshwork, waves, amorphous, and colours. Abnormal appearances and phenomena are also described. Guillon (Tearscope Plus™, 1997) reported the prevalence of LLT for each of these categories as shown in Table 6.5.

Table 6.6 shows the prevalence of LLT in 104 subjects using a custom instrument (Korb et al., 1994).

This study used a custom-designed hemicylindrical broad-spectrum illumination source and slit-lamp microscope. A specific area below the pupil, 2.5 by 5.0 mm, was used to provide a defined area for observation of LLT. Guillon's Tearscope Plus™ technique utilizes a cool white fluorescent source to illuminate interference patterns over almost all of

Table 6.5 Prevalence of lipid layer thickness (Tearscope Plus™, 1997)

Category/lipid patterns	Thickness (nm)	Prevalence (%)
Absent (very rare)	0–13	0.7
Open meshwork (very thin)	13–50	14.8
Closed meshwork (slightly thicker)	13–50	14.6
Wave (flow)	50–70	29.4
Amorphous	80–90	19.6
Colour fringe	Brown = 90–140; blue = 180	17.0
Abnormal	Irregular thickness	3.8

Table 6.6 Prevalence of lipid layer thickness (Korb et al., 1994)

Observed colour	LLT (nm)		Prevalence (%)	
Grey to white	30–60		41	
Grey/yellow	75	11		(Total for
Yellow	90	8		75–105 nm,
Yellow/brown	105	7		26%)
Brown/yellow	120		18	
Brown	135			
Brown/blue	150			
Blue/brown	165		14	
Blue	180			

the corneal surface area and does not consider a specific area for observation of LLT and patterns.

Comparing the two studies for the prevalence of thin lipid layers, Guillon found a 59 per cent prevalence of lipid layers ≤70 nm, while Korb et al. found 52 per cent ≤75 nm. For thicker lipid layers, Guillon found 37 per cent ≥80 nm while Korb et al. found 47 per cent ≥90 nm. Thus, the prevalence of thinner lipid layers ≤75 nm is in the range of 50–60 per cent and the prevalence of thicker lipid layers ≥80–90 nm is 35–50 per cent.

Dynamic aspects of the lipid layer
Although quantitative values and qualitative descriptions are used to characterize the thickness, form and structure of the lipid layer, it is essential to recognize that the lipid layer is not a static, but rather a dynamic film. The lipid layer is thickest slightly above the meniscus and gradually thins from the inferior to central areas of the cornea as it is

pulled upward over the corneal surface by the return movement of the eyelid. This dynamic process is best observed immediately after the upward movement of the eyelid, when colours and a wide variety of patterns, streaks and wave formations may be visible, depending upon the individual characteristics of the lipid layer.

Thin lipid layers are difficult to observe and quantify because of their lack of distinct features. Both Guillon (Tearscope Plus, 1997) and Korb *et al.* (1994) have reported that a uniform lipid layer appearance occurs only when the lipid layer is thin and devoid of colour and obvious features. However, this uniform appearance may be temporarily changed by a blink, particularly if the blink is forceful. A transient patchy appearance of the lipid layer may occur following a blink, but after additional blinks the habitual pattern will return. This is the result of the expression of immature and inspissated material from the meibomian glands, indicating the possibility of meibomian gland dysfunction and obstructed ducts (Korb and Henriquez, 1980).

In contrast to the difficulty in observing thin lipid layers, the interference patterns of thick lipid layers are colourful and readily observed. Thick lipid layers, particularly if > 120 nm, feature multi-coloured horizontal waves starting at the meniscus and extending upward over the inferior third of the cornea. These multi-coloured wave formations may contain two or three colours separated by 0.5 mm or less, indicating that the thickness of the lipid layer is not uniform but varied. In general, the thicker the lipid layer, the greater the variability in thickness. These wave-like patterns frequently change their direction from a horizontal orientation to combinations of arcuate, circular, oblique and vertically orientated waves and streaks over the pupil and superior areas of the cornea. Although some lipid layers are highly coloured over the entire corneal surface, a more usual occurrence is a graduated decrease in colour from the inferior to the superior corneal areas. This indicates that the lipid layer is thicker over the lower portions of the cornea, while the central portion is thinner, often only half of the thickness of the lower portions.

The characteristics and thicknesses of the lipid layer are not absolute findings but rather an evaluation of the range of characteristics of this dynamic film following a particular blink and blink cycle. During the interblink phase the lipid layer slowly thins. In the case of thicker lipid layers, the colours and other features indicative of thickness gradually fade during the interblink phase. Following the next blink, a thicker lipid layer pattern may reform, depending upon the amount of lipid available in the meniscus and/or expressed from the meibomian glands. Partial blinking will not increase LLT or reform those portions of the lipid layer which are not wiped by the blink; the unwiped areas will continue to thin as evidenced by the fading of colours and other features. In the case of thinner lipid layers, their uniform grey or white appearance observed immediately after the blink may change if the interblink period is extended from several seconds to 5–10 s. Streaks and small droplet-like bodies suggestive of break-up patterns appear. With a complete blink the uniform appearance is restored.

Blinking is vital to the lipid layer. Three deliberate, forceful blinks significantly increase the thickness of the lipid layer by a mean of 33 nm for those lipid layers with baseline measurements of 75–150 nm (Korb *et al.*, 1994). For lipid layers with baseline measurements of <75 nm, the mean increase was 19 nm. Bron (1997) has also concluded that the secretion of meibomian oil is aided by blink action. Incomplete blinking or a decrease in blink rate, such as occurs during prolonged periods of close work, reduces lipid secretion (Linton *et al.*, 1961). Thus, blinking has at least two roles relative to the lipid layer. First, complete blinking, particularly if forceful, will augment the expression of lipids from the meibomian glands (Wolff, 1946; Linton *et al.*, 1961; Korb *et al.*, 1994). Secondly, the blink is solely responsible for spreading the lipid across the tear film and the formation of waves and other patterns that provide appropriate optical characteristics for the tear film.

Clinical examination of the lipid layer

Since the only commercially available instrument for the evaluation of the lipid layer is the Tearscope Plus™, the following comments will be directed to the use of this specific instrument. The instrument is easy to use, and the lipid layer is readily observed, particularly if colours or waves are present. The images seen will be unfamiliar unless one has previous experience with lipid layer observation. Refer to the Tearscope Plus™ clinical handbook which contains both colour photographs and descriptions (Tearscope Plus™, 1997).

Simplified approach to lipid layer classification

A simplified clinical approach to the five-category classification of lipid patterns proposed by Guillon (Guillon *et al.*, 1997; Tearscope Plus™, 1997) is to combine the five into three categories as follows:

1. Thick lipid layers, which are highly desirable
2. Average/marginal thickness lipid layers, indicating probable adequate performance
3. Thin lipid layers, suggesting the probability of associated dry eye signs and symptoms.

A suggested clinical classification is shown in Table 6.7.

Table 6.7 Clinical classification of lipid patterns

Category/pattern	LLT (nm)	Implications
Thick lipid layers = colours Blue 150–180 nm Brown/yellow 120–135 nm Yellow/brown 90–105 nm	90–180	• Highly desirable • Thickness ≥120 nm virtually guarantees an optimal tear film, even if stressed
Average/marginal lipid layers = Waves and flow patterns without colour	60–75	• Marginal LLT suggests a marginal tear film • Probably adequate if not stressed • If stressed by environment, vocation, fatigue or contact lenses, dry eye signs and symptoms may result
Thin lipid layers = white to grey	≤50	• Minimal LLT suggests probable dry eye signs and symptoms, which may be present constantly or intermittently • High probability of developing signs and symptoms later in day, if not present early in day • Almost certain probability of developing dry eye signs and symptoms if stressed by environment, vocation, fatigue or contact lenses

Grading

Grading should be made from observations over at least three blink cycles to assure that the grading is representative of the characteristics of the dynamic tear film. With an average or thin LLT, two additional techniques are helpful to complete the analysis and provide a clinically relevant diagnosis:

1. If the baseline LLT is ≤75 nm (no colours visible following the initial observation), direct the patient to blink hard three times. The LLT should increase after these three forceful blinks if the meibomian glands are normal and secreting lipid (Korb *et al.*, 1994). If the LLT does not increase, even momentarily, the probability is that the majority of the meibomian glands are not secreting (due to obstruction, atrophy

and/or the effects of medications), indicating further specific investigation and possible therapy. Thin lipid layers which are improved by forceful blinking suggest partial or infrequent blinking as a contributing causative agent. These situations may benefit from blink training to improve the amplitude and frequency of the blink. If three forceful blinks do not increase LLT, the next step would be to express the meibomian glands with gentle pressure with the thumb and observe the effect upon LLT (Korb *et al.*, 1994). More forceful expression may also be used to determine the severity of the obstruction (Korb and Greiner, 1994; Korb *et al.*, 1994). These findings substantiate a diagnosis of meibomian gland dysfunction and obstructed orifices

2. Observe the lipid layer over the lower areas of the cornea and immediately above the meniscus by moving the Tearscope Plus™ as close as possible to the eye to illuminate the lower areas of the cornea and by directing the patient to look up 10–20°. Evaluate with both normal and forceful blinking. If waves and colours are seen when fixating in the primary position, the lipid layer should be considered average rather than suspect until proven differently.

These findings should be considered in the overall grading and can also determine whether partial blinking or lid closure is a significant factor that requires treatment. If the thickness of the lipid layer on the central and extreme lower portions of the cornea differs, the LLT on the lower portion of the cornea with normal blinking should be used to classify the LLT.

Role of the lower lid in LLT

The anatomical position of the lower lid has a significant effect on LLT. The usual position of the lower lid margin is at the inferior limbus. The lipid layer is thickest slightly above the grey line formed by the lower meniscus. Thus, when the anatomical position of the lower lid is below the inferior limbus, the lipid layer on the central and lower portions of the cornea tends to be thin; if the lower lid margin is above the limbus, the lipid layer tends to be thicker. For any given eye, the LLT is also influenced by the vertical dimension of the interpalpebral aperture. The lipid layer will immediately thicken if the lower lid is slowly raised by manipulation and will return to baseline on the release and return of the lid to its normal position (care should be exercised not to express the meibomian glands). Since the Tearscope Plus™ may not illuminate the extreme lower areas of the ocular surface, observation of the lipid layer over these lower areas usually requires directing fixation upward 10–20°. During the lipid layer evaluation it is important to position the head to ensure that the normal anatomical position of the lower lid is maintained, otherwise the LLT will be altered.

Lipid layer and humidity

Clinicians are aware of the beneficial effects of high ambient levels of humidity for dry eye symptoms and disorders and also for contact lens wearers presenting dry eye symptoms. Korb *et al.* (1996) evaluated whether an increase in periocular humidity would influence the thickness of the lipid layer. Subjects with a thin lipid layer of ≤60 nm were fitted with modified swimming goggles in which one eye was exposed to conditions of high humidity (approximating 100 per cent) and the other eye remained exposed to ambient room conditions (25°C and 40–50 per cent relative humidity) with the following results (Figure 6.1):

- The eye exposed to the high humidity increased significantly in LLT within 5 minutes and reached a maximum increase after 15–20 minutes
- The magnitude of the increase was surprising – the mean increase more than doubled the LLT from ≤60 nm to 120 nm; the eye exposed to ambient room conditions did not increase in LLT
- Upon return to the lower 40–50 per cent humidity environment the LLT decreased, but after 1 hour the eye that had been exposed to the high humidity remained approximately 25 per cent thicker than baseline
- Moderate to total relief of dry eye symptoms was reported during goggle wear and was correlated to the increase in LLT; the improved comfort remained for 1–3 hours following the removal of the goggle.

The exact reasons for this increase in LLT with increased humidity are not known (Korb *et al.*, 1996). It is unlikely that the quantity of meibomian lipid secretion is enhanced with higher humidity. The observed increase in LLT presumably occurs without additional lipid being introduced into the system. Possible reasons include improved spreading of available lipid, increased hydration of the anionic surfactant molecules of the lipid layer, a potential thickening of the aqueous, changes in tear film osmolarity, changes in the solvation state of aqueous macromolecules, or combinations of these factors.

Thus, changes in relative humidity, particularly if large, alter LLT and are an important clinical consideration.

Clinical significance of lipid layer findings

Although many observations of the lipid layer have been reported (Wolff, 1946; Ehlers, 1965; McDonald, 1968; Hamano *et al.*, 1979; Norn, 1979; Guillon, 1982, 1986, 1987; Josephson, 1983; Kilp *et al.*, 1986; Hamano *et al.*, 1992; Guillon and Guillon, 1993; Korb and Greiner, 1994; Korb *et al.*, 1994,

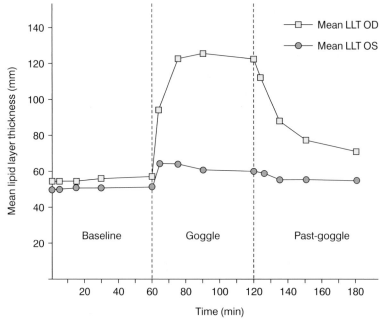

Figure 6.1 Time course of lipid layer thickness changes before, during and after goggle wear. Data points are the mean for the right and left eyes for all subjects. Analysis was made using the paired t test, with a P of <0.01 accepted as significant: baseline, no significant differences; goggle, P<0.0001 for all time points; post-goggle: 5 min, P<0.0001; 15 min, P< 0.0001; 30 min, P<0.001; 60 min, P<0.003

1996; Yokoi *et al.*, 1996; Craig and Tomlinson, 1997; Guillon *et al.*, 1997; Tearscope Plus, 1997), the interpretation of lipid layer findings and their correlation to clinical performance have only recently attracted attention.

In 1997, Craig and Tomlinson established a correlation between the lipid layer, evaporation and tear film stability. They reported that if the lipid layer was minimal or not confluent, tear evaporation was increased four times and the tear film was unstable. Guillon *et al.* (1997) reported that the stability of the tear film was influenced by the nature of the lipid layer, with greater stability being achieved when the lipid layer was thick. They further demonstrated that asymptomatic non-lens wearers had a more stable tear film than symptomatic non-lens wearers. Korb and Greiner (1994) reported that when LLT increased following treatment of meibomian gland dysfunction, symptomatic relief of dry eye symptoms, including discomfort and/or sandy, gritty and foreign-body sensations, was achieved by all subjects. Yokoi *et al.* (1996) found a high correlation between lipid layer patterns and the diagnosis of dry eye severity using seven other tests.

Isreb *et al.* (In press) found that if the LLT was marginal or thin (≤60 nm), the Schirmer and FBUT findings were also depressed (≤5 mm and ≤5 s respectively), indicating aqueous tear deficiency and tear film instability. If the LLT was ≥120 nm, both the Schirmer and FBUT findings indicated optimal tear volume, secretion, and tear film stability. (A rare exception occurs if the lipid layer is highly irregular, beaded, and debris littered, in which case it may be coloured, denoting desirable thickness, but may not be stable. Immature droplets from the meibomian glands may be expressed with blinking, and may create localized areas of increased thickness but with irregular patterns. These problems are most frequently associated with significant blepharitis and meibomitis.) Isreb *et al.*'s findings confirm those of Craig and Tomlinson (1997) and suggest that LLT measurement is an accurate predictor for both the compromised and the optimal tear film.

There are many factors that influence the evaluation and measurement of the lipid layer, including: the ambient humidity; reading or computer use prior to evaluation with associated lipid layer thinning from reduced blinking; diurnal variations; the specific instrumentation and characteristics of the light source used for lipid layer evaluation; the technique of measurement; and the nature of blinking during the diagnostic observation. LLT and all interference pattern observations are the result of optical phenomena and cannot provide direct biochemical information. Care must be taken to ensure that interpretation of the findings is made after considering all of the variables and the established facts.

One would expect that lipid layer deficiency would result in lack of protection for the tear film with subsequent staining of the exposed portions of the ocular surfaces. However, Lee and Tseng (1997) reported that preferential distribution of rose bengal staining on the non-exposed areas of the bulbar conjunctiva characterized lipid tear deficiency and further helped differentiate it from aqueous tear deficiency. The diagnosis of lipid tear deficiency was made by transillumination of the meibomian glands and meibography. Interference patterns of the lipid layer and LLT were not evaluated. It will be of interest to observe whether this new finding, while contrary to clinical experience and intuition, will prove to be of clinical significance.

Summary

The lipid layer is a dynamic rather that a static structure and its evaluation should be considered a dynamic rather than a static evaluation.

- The lipid layer is not intended to be of uniform thickness
- Complete blinking, particularly if forceful, promotes secretion and increases LLT

- Lipid layer thickness is correlated to dry eye disorders
- The lipid layer is primarily secreted from the meibomian glands and is observed using interference phenomena; quantification of LLT is achieved by the observation of interference patterns and colours
- A new commercially available instrument for analysis of lipid layer characteristics and LLT, the Tearscope Plus™, provides the practitioner with a new modality for the diagnosis, monitoring, and management of the tear film and dry eye conditions and disorders
- Colours indicate a thick and desirable lipid layer, which is correlated to optimal tear film stability and optimal tear film characteristics
- Waves or flow patterns without colour indicate an average or marginal thickness lipid layer and probable adequate performance in maintaining tear film stability unless stressed
- If only white or shades of grey are observed, the lipid layer is thin; thin lipid layers (≤ 50–$60\,nm$) are correlated with tear film instability, increased evaporation rate, aqueous tear deficiency and dry eye disorders
- The lipid layer is thickest slightly above the grey line of the meniscus of the lower lid and gradually thins from the inferior to the central areas of the cornea, changing with blinking
- The lower areas of the lipid layer, approaching the meniscus, may be examined by directing the patient to look up 10–20° and to blink as usual
- Observation and grading should be made over the course of at least three blinks
- If waves or colours are not visible with habitual blinking, ask the patient to blink hard three times and continue observation.

LLT is correlated to dry eye symptoms, tear film stability, evaporation rate, and aqueous tear deficiency. It also offers a direct and readily administered test to evaluate if meibomian gland secretion is adequate to increase LLT. It would therefore appear that lipid layer evaluation will become an integral part of the clinician's routine diagnostic examination. It should also become a part of the pre-contact lens fitting and subsequent contact lens examination regime of the contact lens practitioner.

Strategy for diagnosis of tear film disorders and dry eyes

Introduction

The relevant question, 'What to do in a busy practice in cases with suspicion of dry eye?' was posed by Norn (1992), but remains without either a universally accepted answer or strategy. More than 40 specific tests have been reported for the evaluation of the tear film, for use in clinical practice or for research, or both. The 1998 survey of 68 practitioners revealed that more than 25 diagnostic tests were used in their everyday practices or research activities. The tests selected by the 68 respondents as their first choice test, if only one test were allowed, in order of preference were:

Test	Respondents' first choice test (%)
History	28
Fluorescein BUT	19
Rose bengal staining	10
Schirmer	8
Slit-lamp examination	7
Fluorescein staining	3
Lissamine green	<3
Meniscus height	<3
Fluorescein clearance	<3
Osmolarity	<3

The goal of this section is to present the background and the information required for the practitioner to develop a clinically feasible, time efficient, history-directed testing routine for the diagnosis of tear film disorders. The author's personal recommendations will also be presented. The time constraints of the practising clinician and the patient obviously prohibit the use of all or even the majority of the available diagnostic tests on a routine basis. Different strategies may be utilized according to the type of practice: primary care, specialty referral, or contact lens.

The selection of a specific test or tests should be based on the most recent information on the tear film, the patient's history, and the test methods best suited to diagnose the probable type of disorder. Practically, the tests utilized by the majority of clinicians are limited to those that can be performed with standard clinical equipment. Further, as reported by Bron (1997), it is important for tests to be carried out in correct sequence and at the appropriate intervals, in order to avoid one test interfering with the other.

While it is clear that there is no one universal first choice test for the evaluation of the tear film and the detection of tear film disorders, the comments of the survey respondents and a review of the literature establish that tear film stability and osmolarity are the two common denominator findings associated with virtually all dry eye states (Gilbard and Farris, 1979; Gilbard, 1994; Pflugfelder et al., 1998). If accurate, reliable, and clinically feasible tests for these two tear film characteristics were available, the diagnosis of a tear film disorder could readily be made, although these two end-point findings would not provide the specific cause of the disorder. Because of the importance of osmolarity and tear film stability, their strategic use in the diagnosis of tear film disorders will be reviewed.

Osmolarity

The osmolarity of the tears is not readily measured in routine clinical practice since it requires specialized instrumentation and is difficult to perform accurately. A new clinical osmometer (Nanoliter Osmometer, Model 3000, Advanced Instruments Inc., U.S.A.) has been reported to provide reproducible data without highly skilled operators (Awad *et al.*, 1998) and to be more functional than other osmometers for office-based testing (Foulks *et al.*, 1998). Further experience with this instrument along with future technological development will determine whether osmolarity measurement will remain a secondary test (Lemp, 1995), limited to research use, or whether it will become a part of primary and/or tertiary practice.

Tear film stability

The tests used to evaluate tear film stability are fluorescein break-up time (FBUT) or non-invasive break-up time (NIBUT). While NIBUT presents an ideal theoretical model to measure tear film stability, it probably will not replace FBUT as the first choice test in the near future. The reader is referred to the section on tear film stability and BUT for a complete understanding of the relevant issues and techniques for FBUT and NIBUT.

If an unstable tear film is, as reported by Pflugfelder *et al.* (1998), 'the hallmark of various dry-eye states', it would appear that the FBUT test should be a critical component of tear film diagnosis. However, the controversy concerning the clinical relevance of the FBUT test is borne out by the survey's 68 respondents, only 19 per cent of whom reported FBUT as their first choice test and only 50 per cent of whom used FBUT as one of their four routine preferred tests. The reported reasons for the lack of acceptance of the standard FBUT test were its inaccuracy, lack of scientific base, and failure to provide reproducible data (Marquardt *et al.*, 1986; Mengher *et al.*, 1985b, 1986; Larke, 1997).

The accuracy and reproducibility of the FBUT test have been reported to increase when the volume of fluorescein instilled is reduced to 2 µl or less by utilizing an ultra micro digital pipette (Marquardt *et al.*, 1986). This technique is obviously not readily adaptable to routine clinical practice. The interested practitioner may modify existing methods and techniques for the application of the fluorescein, as described in the section on tear stability and FBUT, and achieve improved accuracy and reproducibility for FBUT findings, the limiting factor being the ability to control the volume of fluorescein applied to the eye. It is essential for the clinician to have confidence in his or her method of diagnosis of tear film stability, one of the global end-points and hallmarks of dry eye states.

Recognizing the need for controlling the volume of fluorescein delivered, Korb *et al.* (1999) reported a new fluorescein strip method for the FBUT test, which allows the delivery of 1 µl of fluorescein solution. FBUT measurement may be made immediately, without the usual 60 s wait, and with comparable accuracy and reproducibility to that achieved by the delivery of 1 µl of fluorescein by the pipette method. This new strip is marketed as the DET test by Akorn Inc., Buffalo, Illinois.

History

History is a critical tool in the diagnosis of tear film disorders, especially if the condition is intermittent or varying in intensity. History was reported as the first choice test by the 68 respondents in the 1998 survey, confirming its importance to both clinicians and researchers. Lowther (1997) credits history as the most important test in diagnosing a marginal dry eye patient.

The report of the National Eye Institute/industry workshop and clinical trials on dry eyes considered symptoms, which are elicited through the history, as one of the four global tests for dry eye (Lemp, 1995). The history should include not only ocular symptoms, but also general systemic conditions, allergies, and both over-the-counter and prescription medications, which may cause dry eye symptoms.

The history can be obtained by verbal questioning, written questionnaires, or a combination of the two.

Verbal questioning

Verbal questioning has been the traditional method of obtaining information and will usually reveal complaints and symptoms. Questioning establishes a dialogue and an interactive relationship between the examiner and the patient. It allows the assessment of the relative importance and magnitude of symptoms as well as assisting the examiner in establishing a hypothesis for the most likely causes of the reported problems. Adequate time must be allowed to pursue questioning, particularly if patients are inhibited in their responses or fail to differentiate between responding and complaining. The examiner must recognize the tendency for some patients to consider their symptoms as 'normal' and/or an unavoidable part of the ageing process or specific compromising activities, such as prolonged computer use, and therefore may not report their presence.

Written questionnaire

Written questionnaires have the obvious advantage of presenting standardized questions without consuming professional time. Several excellent, validated questionnaires are available and have been presented in the chapter by Guillon. They have been advocated for use with:

- The entire adult population, since it is commonly believed that adults of all ages can suffer from dry eye (Schein et al., 1996)
- Adult women, since dry eye is more common with women than men (Jacobsen et al., 1989)
- The elderly, although the data for prevalence among the elderly is inconclusive (Strickland et al., 1987; Schein et al., 1996)
- Certain environments and occupations which are reported to result in dry eye symptoms (Korb, 1994)
- Contact lens wearers, since contact lenses can provoke dry eye symptoms and cause the contact lens-induced dry eye (McMonnies and Ho, 1986; Tomlinson, 1992)
- Contact lens candidates, with questioning directed towards detecting marginal dry eye symptoms prior to the fitting of contact lenses (Lowther, 1997).

The questionnaire chosen by the examiner will vary with the type of practice and the goals of the examiner. Two excellent questionnaires for general practice have been developed by McMonnies and Ho and by Rolando et al. (1998), while a more specific contact lens-oriented questionnaire may be preferable for screening the contact lens candidate or wearer (McMonnies and Ho, 1986, 1987; Lowther, 1993, 1997; Rolando et al., 1998).

Combined verbal questioning and written questionnaire

Many clinicians prefer to utilize a written questionnaire as a starting point and follow-up with verbal questioning, as indicated, to develop a more comprehensive understanding of the patient's situation. This combination offers the optimal subjective method for detecting and understanding the nature of possible tear film disorders. It will frequently reveal not only the symptoms but possible related causes. Appropriate questioning by the examiner will help to establish the frequency and magnitude of the problem and to determine the specific tests required for diagnosis.

Symptoms

The most common symptoms reported by dry eye patients are a sandy, gritty feeling, soreness and scratchiness (Holly, 1989). If KCS is present, dryness and grittiness are the dominant symptoms (McMonnies and Ho, 1987). Other reported symptoms include heaviness of the lids, foreign-body sensation, discomfort associated with blink actions, stinging, photophobia, and the paradoxical tearing and/or watering resulting from irritation. These symptoms have been clinically associated with dry eye states and the work of McMonnies and Ho (1987) has validated this association.

However, according to Norn (1992), a patient with dry eyes may not necessarily report these symptoms, since they may not recognize them as such or may simply endure mild to moderate discomfort which they assume to be normal. Patients may report general ocular symptoms such as heaviness or visual or ocular fatigue especially at the end of the day, which can be a symptom of dry eye, but which may not be recognized as a dry eye symptom by the clinician. While it is acknowledged that dry eye usually causes symptoms, in some patients in whom a diagnosis of dry eye is strongly suggested on the basis of signs, symptoms could be absent (Lemp, 1995).

The more severe the dry eye condition, the greater the probability of significant discomfort and/or pain. Severe episodes of pain should alert the practitioner to the possibility of recurrent corneal erosion, particularly if the pain is episodic or tends to occur upon awakening. This may or may not be associated with dry eye states, but diagnosis is essential for effective treatment.

Whenever symptoms suggestive of dry eye are present from the history, the practitioner should assume that dry eye exists until proven differently and the appropriate testing should be carried out. In the ideal hypothetical situation a given eye would exhibit a steady state of tear film disorder, independent of diurnal variation, ambient environment, occupation, physical condition, influence of medication, visual demands and fatigue. This is obviously not the case and the practitioner must recognize that symptoms deserve further consideration, even when certain objective tests fail to reveal an anomaly on a given day.

Clinical strategy

The ultimate goal of the evaluation of the patient with dry eye symptoms is to determine the cause or causes of the tear film disorder and then to provide effective treatment, which, as pointed out by Pflugfelder *et al.* (1998), is dependent on an accurate diagnosis and matching the treatment to the diagnosis. These authors also acknowledged the importance of recognizing that the cause of dry eye states may be multifactorial. The strategy for the evaluation should be directed to selecting the specific tests and the sequence of testing to achieve these goals.

Pflugfelder et al. *and Bron sequences of testing*

Two excellent strategies and procedures for the selection of the tests and the sequence of testing for dry eye disorders have been presented by Pflugfelder *et al.* (1998) and by Bron (1997). Both are valuable contributions because they detail specific procedures and the sequence of testing. The sequence of testing and the appropriate time intervals between tests

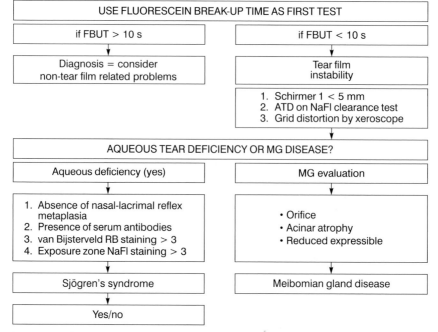

Figure 6.2 Sequence of testing symptoms of ocular irritation (modified from Pflugfelder *et al.*, 1998)

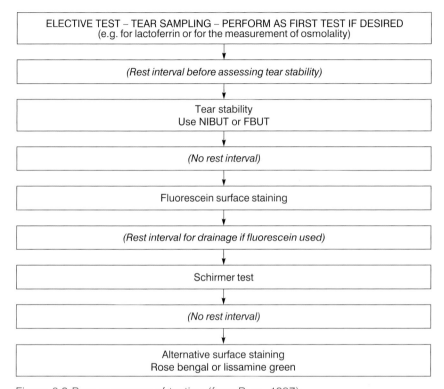

Figure 6.3 Bron sequence of testing (from Bron, 1997)

are important considerations because of the effects of each test on those that follow. An obvious example would be conducting the Schirmer test following the use of fluorescein, which might add additional fluid volume to the eye. If the sequence of testing is not carefully considered, there is a significant probability that one or more of the test results will be erroneous and might even be misleading.

The Pflugfelder *et al.* and Bron sequences of testing are summarized in Figures 6.2 and 6.3.

FBUT role in strategy of testing

Both Pflugfelder *et al.* (1998) and Bron (1997) attribute a primary role to the FBUT test. Pflugfelder *et al.* utilized the FBUT test to determine if symptoms of ocular irritation were tear film related, with values >10 s

Dry Eye Survey

Please answer the following by indicating the response most appropriate to you.

Age:	Under 25 years	25 – 45 years	Over 45 years

Currently wearing:	No contact lenses	Hard contact lenses	Soft contact lenses

1 Do you ever experience any of the following eye symptoms? *Please underline those that apply to you*

Soreness	Scratchiness	Dryness	Grittiness	Burning

2 How often do your eyes have these symptoms?

Never	Sometimes	Often	Constantly

3 Have you ever had drops prescribed or other treatment for dry eyes?

Yes	No	Uncertain

4 Do you suffer from arthritis?

Yes	No	Uncertain

5 Do you suffer from thyroid abnormality?

Yes	No	Uncertain

6 Do you experience dryness of the nose, mouth, throat, chest or vagina?

Never	Sometimes	Often	Constantly

7 Do you regard your eyes as being unusually sensitive to cigarette smoke, smog, air conditioning, central heating?

Yes	No	Sometimes

8 Do your eyes easily become very red and irritated when swimming in chlorinated fresh water?

Not applicable	Yes	No	Sometimes

9 Do you take or use any of the following?

Antihistamine tablets	Antihistamine eye drops	Diuretics (fluid tablets)	Sleeping tablets
Tranquillizers	Oral contraceptives	Sleeping tablets	
Medication for duodenal ulcer or digestive problems or for high blood pressure			

Other
(please write) _____

10 Are your eyes dry and irritated the day after drinking alcohol?

Not applicable	Yes	No	Sometimes

11 Are you known to sleep with your eyes partly open?

Yes	No	Sometimes

12 Do you have eye irritation as you wake from sleep?

Yes	No	Sometimes

Figure 6.4 McMonnies questionnaire

Dry Eye Survey

System of Scoring Responses:

Male or female	under 25 years	0
Male	25–45 years	1
Female	25–45 years	3
Male	over 45 years	2
Female	over 45 years	6

Question 2 – frequency of primary symptoms:

Never	0
Sometimes	1
Often	4
Constantly	8

Question 3 – previous treatment:

Yes	6
No or uncertain	0

Question 4 – arthritis:

Yes	2
No or uncertain	0

Question 5 – thyroid abnormality:

Yes	2
No or uncertain	0

Question 6 – mucous membrane dryness:

Never	0
Sometimes	1
Often	2
Constantly	4

Question 7 – unusual sensitivity:

No	0
Sometimes	2
Yes	4

Question 8 – swimming irritation:

Not applicable and no	0
Sometimes	1
Yes	2

Question 9 – medication side effect:

Antihistamine tablets or eye drops or diuretics	2
Sleeping tablets or tranquillizers or oral contraceptives, duodenal ulcer/digestive/high blood preeure medication	1

Question 10 – alcohol:

Not applicable or no	0
Sometimes	2
Yes	4

Question 11 – nocturnal lagophthalmos:

Not applicable or no	0
Sometimes	1
Yes	2

Question 12 – waking irritation:

No	0
Sometimes	1
Yes	2

The grading for the McMonnies questionnaire may be summarized as follows (McMonnies et al., 1998):

Normal	0–9
Marginal dry eye	10–20
Dry eye	>20

Figure 6.4 continued

indicating non-tear film related problems and values < 10 s indicating tear film instability and the probable presence of a dry eye disorder. According to this strategy, if the FBUT were > 10 s, despite the presence of symptoms of ocular irritation, the tear film investigation would be terminated and non-tear film related problems would be considered.

The initial task is to establish the diagnosis of a dry eye and, having made that diagnosis, to determine the cause. The FBUT test can serve as the first step in dry eye diagnosis, provided the examiner has confidence that the FBUT test as administered in his or her hands is accurate and reproducible.

If the FBUT finding is clearly abnormally low (5 s or less), the diagnosis of dry eye is established (Mackie and Seal, 1981). Break-up times of 5–10 s are considered to be marginal for dry eye (Tomlinson, 1992), but this diagnosis should be confirmed by repeating the FBUT test on another day. Lowther (1997) reported that many patients with break-up times in the 8–10 s range (or even less) may be successful contact lens wearers, despite the additional stress on the tear film created by contact lenses, thereby suggesting that the 8–10 s range may not always be diagnostic. If the FBUT is > 10 s, there is a high probability that the eye is not dry. The accuracy and reproducibility of the FBUT measurement is essential to any diagnosis; obviously, misdiagnosis will result if the FBUT values are erroneous.

Author's strategy and procedure for diagnosis of tear film disorders

A history to determine the presence of symptoms associated with dry eye disorder is invaluable and should precede diagnostic testing. The McMonnies questionnaire is recommended and is reproduced in Figure 6.4. A supplementary questionnaire for relevant medications and systemic conditions is provided in Figure 6.5.

Sequence of tests

The author's sequence of testing is provided in Figure 6.6. The tests may be discontinued at any point in the sequence when the findings establish or negate the diagnosis of dry eye. If desired, additional tests are conducted to determine the cause of the dry eye disorder.

The initial approach is to utilize non-invasive tests which will not influence subsequent tests. The two recommended tests are the biomicroscopic evaluation of the lids and ocular surfaces and lipid layer

Dry Eye Survey

**Medications and systemic diseases that can affect
the tear film and cause dry eye symptoms**

Tick all that apply

Medications

- Antibiotics . . . . □
- Tetracycline . . . . □
- Antihistamines . . . . □
- Allergy medications . . . . □
- Sinus medications . . . . □
- Sleep medications . . . . □
- Diet medications . . . . □
- Antihypertensives . . . . □
- Methyldopate hydrochloride . . . . □
- Reserpine . . . . □
- Antiperspirants (long-term) . . . . □
- Belladonna alkaloids. . . . . □
- Bellergal. . . . . □
- Donnatal . . . . □
- Pro-Banthine . . . . □
- B-Blockers (topical) . . . . □
- Birth control medications . . . . □
- Botulinum toxin . . . . □
- Dermatologic medications . . . . □
- Isotretinoin. . . . . □
- Diuretics . . . . □
- Chlorothiazides . . . . □
- Furosemide . . . . □
- Hydrochlorothiazide . . . . □
- Hormones . . . . □
- Oral contraceptives . . . . □
- Psychotomimetics . . . . □
- Chlordiazepoxide . . . . □
- Diazepam. . . . . □
- Amitriptyline. . . . . □
- Thioridazine . . . . □

Systemic conditions

- Connective tissue diseases . . . . □
- Hormone disorders . . . . □
- Mucous tissue dryness . . . . □
- Rheumatic diseases. . . . . □
- Thyroid . . . . □

Figure 6.5 Supplementary questionnaire (modified from Lowther, 1997 and Rolando *et al.*, 1998)

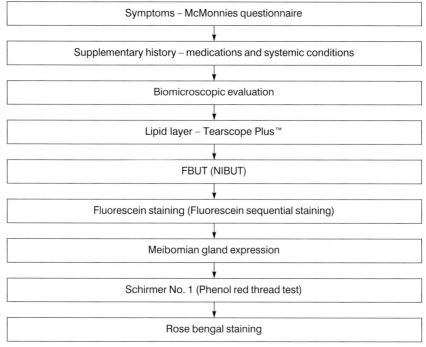

Figure 6.6 Korb sequence of testing

evaluation with interference patterns if instrumentation is available. (The NIBUT test is not recommended at this time since instrumentation for this evaluation is not available.)

Following these non-invasive tests, the break-up time test is conducted with the addition of fluorescein. If the biomicroscopic evaluation is negative, the LLT > 90 nm, and the FBUT > 10 s, further testing may not be indicated (Pflugfelder *et al.*, 1998; Isreb *et al.*, in press).

Corneal and conjunctival staining may be assessed immediately upon conclusion of the FBUT test. If micro amounts of sodium fluorescein are utilized for the FBUT test, additional fluorescein is required to disclose the full extent of the epithelial staining. If desired, fluorescein sequential staining may also be carried out at this time. Meibomian gland expression is the next step and may be performed between sequential instillations of fluorescein. Meibomian gland expression may reveal meibomian gland dysfunction, which may be the cause of either an existing or imminent tear film disorder which cannot be diagnosed in any other manner. The author includes meibomian gland expression whenever there are symptoms or any indications of a dry eye disorder or when there are any symptoms with contact lens wearers.

Prior to conducting the Schirmer test, excess fluid resulting from the FBUT and fluorescein staining tests must be eliminated, requiring a rest period or returning on another day. An alternative is to blot the excess tears using the method described in the author's procedure for the Schirmer test. Rose bengal staining should be scheduled as the last test because of the possible discomfort, induced reflex tearing, and surface alterations which could necessitate a long recovery period prior to conducting other tear film tests. In all but the most unusual circumstances, the sequence of tests from history to rose bengal staining provides a comprehensive evaluation and may be conducted at one extended visit if adequate time is available.

The following specialized tests are considered research tests and are not usually performed in routine clinical practice: fluorescein clearance (retention) tests, tear proteins, osmolarity, evaporation, impression cytology, immunologic testing, and reflex tearing.

Mackie and Seal (1981) addressed the problem of recognition and diagnosis of the 'questionably dry eye', which was defined as not a severely dry eye, but an eye with at least one feature of dryness in a patient with symptoms suggestive of dryness. They found that the diagnosis of the questionably dry eye could best be made by the tear lysozyme test. However, this test is currently not in widespread clinical use.

Biomicroscopic evaluation

Routine biomicroscopic examination of the external lids, lid margins, meibomian glands, inferior tear meniscus, tear film and debris, blink and lid closure should be conducted as the first test following history because it is non-invasive and does not alter the eye or influence the other tests. This examination should not employ physical manipulation of the lids; a 'look but no touch' approach should be used to avoid influencing the tests that follow.

The lids should be specifically examined for those conditions which are known to be correlated with or are a cause of dry eye disorders or dry eye symptoms. These include:

- Inflammation of the external lids
- Ectropion or incomplete apposition of the lower lid margin to the ocular surfaces
- Blepharitis, including desquamation and/or scaling of the skin and/or collarettes around the base of the lashes
- Tear film characteristics related to debris and mucous strands in the tear film
- Lower lid margin irregularity
- Dried mucoid material adhering to the lower lid margin

- Injection and/or hyperaemia of the bulbar conjunctiva
- Foam along the lid margins, but more commonly appearing on the skin at the temporal canthus
- Meibomian gland orifice abnormalities
- Incomplete lid closure.

Diffuse inflammation of the lids or lid margins and/or signs of blepharitis directly suggest tear film difficulties and surface problems involving the lower aspects of the cornea as reported by McCulley and Sciallis (1977) and Abelson (1983). There is also a high prevalence of significant meibomian gland dysfunction with these conditions.

Tear film debris or excess mucus suggests a tear volume problem, usually aqueous deficiency, particularly when accompanied by dried mucoid material on the lid margins.

Foam is frequently overlooked during the examination; however, it is a remarkably reliable indicator of meibomian gland dysfunction (MGD) and should be considered indicative of some level of MGD until proven differently (Korb and Henriquez, 1980).

Normal meibomian gland orifices appear as closed or half-closed openings. The orifices have been described as surrounded by a white mother-of-pearl-like matrix, more transparent than the neighbouring tissues (Berliner, 1949). The orifices should be evaluated for distension or pouting caused by internal secretion in the underlying duct, protruding material in the form of filaments, the presence of foam or bubbles adhering on the tissue immediately surrounding the orifice, and epithelial overgrowth over the orifices. The overgrowth of epithelium may actually prevent observation of the orifice. Meibomian gland orifice abnormalities indicate MGD, which should be further investigated by expression conducted after the break-up time test.

Lid closure may be evaluated during the biomicroscopic examination by passing the slit beam over the closed lids and observing the completeness of the closure. Lid closure is frequently incomplete nasally, but complete along the remainder of the lid margins. Incomplete closure may result in compromise to the inferior corneal and conjunctival surfaces.

Lipid layer evaluation

Lipid layer evaluation may be performed before or following biomicroscopy (as the first or second test, depending upon convenience), because it is non-invasive and does not alter the eye or influence the other tests. This evaluation requires specialized instrumentation. The only commercially available instrument is the Tearscope Plus™ (Tearscope Plus™, 1997). With this instrument, lipid layer evaluation is readily performed within 60–120 s. Because lipid layer thickness (LLT) is correlated to dry eye disorders, it promises to become an important test in establishing the presence of dry eye disorders.

Since the lipid layer is reviewed in detail in the preceding section, only a synopsis of clinically relevant considerations for this test will be included at this time:

1. Care must be taken to direct the patient to blink before classifying the observed pattern, since the LLT may decrease between blinks, especially if the inter-blink period is > 10 s. Evaluate LLT over the course of three blinks
2. If the LLT on the central areas of the cornea is less than 90 nm, instruct the patient to 'blink hard three times', and use this observation to classify the LLT
3. If the lipid layer thickness on the central areas of the cornea remains < 90 nm after the three forceful blinks, the lower areas of the lipid layer starting approximately 1 mm above the meniscus should be evaluated. This is accomplished by directing fixation 10–20° superiorly, asking the patient to blink hard three times, and then observing the resulting lipid layer characteristics and patterns on the lower portion of the eye. Consider this finding in classifying LLT.

The lipid layer characteristics should be interpreted as follows:

● The appearance of colours indicates a thick and desirable lipid layer and suggests that dry eye disorder is not present (blue = 150–180 nm, red/brown = 120–35 nm, yellow = 90–105 nm)
● Waves or flow patterns without pronounced colours, especially if horizontal, indicate an average or marginal thickness lipid layer, and possible mild dry eye disorder (75 nm)
● If only white or shades of grey (particularly if the white or grey is uniform) are observed, the lipid layer is thin (≤60 nm) and the probability of a dry eye disorder is high.

As a practical consideration, the design of the Tearscope Plus™ allows it to be conveniently mounted on the applanation tonometer post of the slit lamp and swings into place in the same way as the applanation tonometer. A limitation, however, is that only one instrument can be mounted and used at one time.

Break-up time
NIBUT
While NIBUT measurement would appear to offer an ideal theoretical method to assess tear film stability, it has not achieved general clinical acceptance. Pflugfelder et al. (1998) reported that the longer NIBUT with

a normal range of 40–60 s and the shorter 10–30 s FBUT evaluate different phenomena and, therefore, the NIBUT would not replace the FBUT test. Unless the clinician has appropriate instrumentation and significant experience with the NIBUT test, the author concurs with Pflugfelder's conclusion.

FBUT

The FBUT test should be employed to evaluate tear film stability. The FBUT has been summarized in this section and a complete review was provided in a preceding section. The reader is referred to this section.

Fluorescein staining

Evaluation of fluorescein staining may be made immediately after the FBUT test, observing the staining produced by the fluorescein instilled for the FBUT test. If the amount of fluorescein used for the FBUT test is < 5 μl, it may be inadequate to allow optimal corneal and conjunctival staining, requiring the instillation of additional fluorescein prior to the evaluation of staining. Sequential fluorescein staining may be conducted with additional instillations of fluorescein. The reader is referred to the preceding section on ocular surface staining for a detailed discussion of fluorescein staining.

Meibomian gland expression

The routine biomicroscopic examination of the external lids includes evaluation of the lid margins and meibomian gland orifices. If inflammation is present about the orifices of the glands and on the margins of the lids, the meibomian glands are usually affected and meibomitis is present.

The term meibomian gland dysfunction was introduced by Korb and Henriquez (1980) to describe a syndrome characterized by deficient or inadequate meibomian gland secretion due to obstruction of the ducts of the meibomian glands by keratotic plugs, but frequently without the obvious inflammatory and other characteristic external signs occurring with meibomitis. The typical forms of meibomitis are readily diagnosed by external signs including: inflammation, vascularization, thickening, and serration of the lid margins; pouting and abnormal material extending from the orifices; foam on the lid margins and/or menisci, and deposition of oil droplets and abnormal waxy material on the lid margins. (Blepharitis usually accompanies meibomitis, particularly the more severe forms, as with meibomian keratoconjunctivitis (McCulley and Sciallis, 1977).) Expression of glands with meibomitis may provide varied results, from no secretion despite the application of extreme pressure, suggesting total blockage of the ducts, to grossly excessive amounts of inspissated secretion.

In contrast, MGD may not be obvious, since the external signs may be absent or so minimal that they are overlooked. The external signs of MGD are frequently limited to subtle alterations of the meibomian orifices, incipient overgrowth of epithelium over the orifices, and foam, most often on the skin at the temporal canthi. Since the external signs required for diagnosis of MGD may not be present, the condition is frequently not recognized. The diagnosis of MGD requires evaluating whether the meibomian glands yield normal secretion or whether the ducts are obstructed, resulting in deficient or altered secretion. The delivery of meibomian gland secretion to the tear film during the waking state is aided by blink action, an observation which was first reported by Wolff over 50 years ago, and has subsequently been studied by numerous investigators (Wolff, 1946; Linton et al., 1961; McDonald, 1968; Korb et al., 1994; Bron, 1997). Since the minimal pressure of blinking is adequate to express secretion from the meibomian glands, evaluation of whether a gland is normal and secreting or partially or totally obstructed requires a similar amount of pressure applied to the gland while observation is made with the biomicroscope.

To evaluate the status of the meibomian glands and the possibility of MGD in the absence of significant signs, the following procedure is recommended:

1. Observe the central third of the lower lid margin, selecting six to eight meibomian gland orifices for study
2. Gently express the meibomian glands in this area with the thumb against the lower lid surface to obtain secretions
3. If no secretion is obtained with gentle pressure, repeat the expression with increased pressure using the same technique
4. Forceful expression may be performed by grasping the lid between the index finger and the thumb, or by compressing the meibomian glands between the thumb on the external lid surface and a Q-tip or rigid object placed against the corresponding palpebral surface of the lid after topical anaesthesia. The diagnostic value of forceful expression is to determine whether a gland will yield secretion. Forceful expression is also a part of MGD treatment (Korb and Greiner, 1994)
5. If upon mild pressure all of the orifices yield minute amounts of clear fluid, the glands are normal (Berliner, 1949) and MGD is not present. If all of the orifices, in the absence of significant signs, do not yield any secretion despite forceful pressure, the ducts are totally obstructed (or atrophied) and MGD is present. Other findings are more difficult to classify, since the classification involves the ratio of the glands which

yield secretion versus those which are obstructed, the nature of the expressed secretion and the magnitude of the pressure which is applied.

The following classification of MGD (in the absence of significant signs) has been found to be helpful in the author's practice:

Normal or optimal	Clear fluid is expressed with gentle pressure from 75 per cent or more of the orifices; if the expressed secretion is not clear, the status is not optimal
Mild MGD	Clear or milky fluid is expressed from 50 per cent or more of the orifices with gentle pressure
Moderate MGD	One or both of the following are present:

- Less than 50 per cent of the orifices yield any type of secretion with gentle or increased pressure
- The secretion is inspissated or creamy, resembling pus. Inspissated secretion may be expressed in a number of forms including fine filamentary, columnar resembling expressed toothpaste, and more globular forms. These forms are not diagnostic, but probably result from the nature of the obstruction of the duct and the orifice

Severe MGD   One or both of the following are present:

- Less than 75 per cent of the orifices yield any type of secretion with gentle or increased pressure
- The inspissated secretion appears purulent, suggesting the presence of bacteria

Summary
- MGD may not present obvious external signs, and may therefore not be recognized
- Expression of the glands is required to diagnose MGD and to determine if their secretion is optimal, compromised, or whether the ducts are obstructed. Total obstruction of the ducts may be present resulting in no secretion.

The Schirmer test

The measurement of tear production is considered an essential finding in the diagnosis of dry eye (Mackie and Seal, 1981; Abelson and Lamberts,

1983). The classical method for measuring tear production was introduced in 1903 by Schirmer (Murube, 1992), but it was not until 1941 when Whatman 41 filter paper was used to standardize the procedure that the test became widely used (de Rötth, 1941). The original procedure was performed with the eyes open and was intended to measure reflex tear production as the result of conjunctival stimulation and blinking. The problems with the Schirmer measurement have long been recognized, as reported by the noted ophthalmologist Sjögren, who in 1950 wrote: 'The lacrimal test of Schirmer is an inexact method, even if it is performed strictly according to the rules' (Norn, 1974).

Modifications have been made to improve the Schirmer test, including conducting the test with the eyes closed (Henderson and Prough, 1950), after topical ocular anaesthesia (Jones, 1966), with papers designed to minimize evaporation (Holly et al., 1986) and with various threads to minimize the sensation (Kurihashi et al., 1977; Kurihashi, 1986). Despite these efforts, the Schirmer test continues to be the subject of numerous criticisms primarily directed to the variability of the findings and the difficulties in standardization (Clinch et al., 1983).

The test without anaesthesia has been criticized as being variable because of the sensation and/or irritation to the eye resulting in unpredictable and/or excess reflex tearing. The Schirmer test may be performed with anaesthesia, but this is also subject to criticism. Jones (1966) suggested using topical anaesthesia when performing the Schirmer test to eliminate reflex tearing, but recognized that the topical anaesthetic would cause irritation and recommended a waiting period prior to measurement. Another factor influencing the Schirmer measurement is the presence of reflex tear secretion despite the use of anaesthesia (Jordan and Baum, 1980). Jones (1966) reported that if the test with topical anaesthesia is conducted with the eyes open, the value is higher than with the anaesthetized eyes closed. Mackie and Seal (1981) also reported that closure of the eyes could result in a false-positive Schirmer finding. The fact that tear production ceases during general anaesthesia has been used to argue that all tear production is the result of stimulation.

It is therefore not surprising that Norn (1992) concluded that anaesthesia should not be used in the Schirmer test, since some tear reflex is in any case unavoidable. The members of the National Eye Institute/industry workshop on clinical trials in dry eyes recommended the Schirmer test without anaesthetic as a better measure of the capacity of the lacrimal glands to produce tears than if an anaesthetic were used (Lemp, 1995).

In addition to the question of using an anaesthetic, precisely what is measured by the Schirmer test is controversial. The original intent was to measure the lacrimal gland tear production rate. This rate may be considered as either basal or reflex secretion, a differentiation initially proposed by Jones (1966). The basal rate is that measured on the anaesthetized eye, supposedly without the contribution of reflex tearing. There are, however, significant data to suggest that the Schirmer test on the anaesthetized eye does not measure so-called basal tear secretion and that basal tear secretion may not be a valid concept (Clinch *et al.*, 1983). The values of the Schirmer test are approximately 40 per cent lower with anaesthesia, a fact used to support the concept of a lower basal tear secretion (Lamberts *et al.*, 1978). There is also the question of the amount of the contribution of the existing tears in the meniscus to the wetting of the strip. The meniscus holds approximately 3 μl of the total tear volume, which averages 7 μl; thus, over 40 per cent of the total tear volume is in the meniscus.

Nelson (1994) reported that the filter strip used for the Schirmer test, even with anaesthesia, undergoes a rapid initial wetting phase due to the absorption of the tear reservoir. After the first 1–2 minutes the wetting of the strip becomes less rapid and more linear. This would suggest that the Schirmer finding is the result of the volume of the tear meniscus, reflex tearing, and tear production. If an anaesthetic is used, the excess fluid should be removed from the meniscus, otherwise the Schirmer finding will be inflated by the residual fluid in the meniscus. This may be accomplished by blotting, or possibly by waiting. Abelson and Lamberts (1983) described the Schirmer test as 'notoriously variable and fraught with sources of error' and suggested repeating it after a 2-minute wait to eliminate tear fluid when using an anaesthetic. Known as the 'double-void technique', this may more accurately reflect tear production.

The inconsistencies in methodology, the basic variability of the test and the question of what is actually measured have led many authors to conclude that any type of Schirmer test is of very little or no clinical value. A sample of recent quotations follows: 'Numerous studies have shown Schirmer test to be unreliable and of little clinical value' (Hom and Shovlin, 1997); 'A frequently quoted but unreliable procedure' (Gasson and Morris, 1998); and 'It is not a very good test for a marginal dry eye that creates the problems with normal contact lens wear' (Lowther, 1997).

Despite these comments, a philosophy presented by Abelson and co-workers requires consideration. Abelson and Lamberts (1983) advised using topical anaesthetic for the Schirmer test, but noted that the use of anaesthetic remained a controversial issue. Abelson and Welch (1994) reported that while the Schirmer test is probably the least reliable of all dry eye tests, if the finding is < 5 mm, there is reason to suspect aqueous deficiency. The author concurs with their analysis that the Schirmer finding is diagnostic if < 5 mm, indicating a deficiency of tear production and/or volume.

Despite its inadequacies, the Schirmer test remains the universal test for the evaluation of the production of tears by the lacrimal glands. The only other Schirmer-like test is the cotton thread test, which requires only 15 s for wetting, causes less irritation and is thought to be an indication of tear volume (Kurihashi et al., 1977; Kurihashi, 1986). This test is available as the Zone-Quick, distributed by Menicon Co., Ltd. While the use of this cotton thread test is increasing, further studies and experience are required before it can substitute for the Schirmer test.

An improved test to measure tear production or tear volume or both, which requires reliable measurement of micro amounts of fluid, is a challenging technical requirement further complicated by the need to either eliminate or standardize sensation and reflex tearing. The current estimates of tear volume and tear flow have been determined by research techniques, primarily using fluorescein and fluorophotometry (Mishima et al., 1966). It would therefore appear that the clinical measurement of tear production and tear volume will not be possible in the immediate future by any method other than the current Schirmer test or its modifications.

Summary and recommendations

Despite remaining an 'inexact method' some 50 years after Sjögren's comment, the Schirmer test provides a highly probable diagnosis of an aqueous-deficient eye if the value is ≤ 5 mm. If the value is ≤ 3 mm, the diagnosis of an aqueous-efficient eye is confirmed. Although one could consider values between 6 mm and the usual cut-off value of 10 mm (or even 15 mm) as in a marginal or grey zone of aqueous deficiency, this zone is best considered inconclusive in ruling out the aqueous-deficient dry eye, since there can be no assurance that an abnormal level of reflex tearing did not occur due to the irritation of the paper strip. Although the same argument can be made with values > 15 mm, the probability of an aqueous-deficient eye with values > 15 mm, in the absence of significant reported sensation during the test, is obviously greatly diminished. Thus, the Schirmer test has the potential to diagnose aqueous deficiency if reflex tearing does not occur, but there can be no assurance that reflex tearing will not inflate the finding and result in misdiagnosis.

Since the primary problem with the Schirmer test without anaesthesia is the variability of stimulation resulting in an unknown level of reflex tearing, the author recommends the use of anaesthetic to minimize the irritation associated with the presence of the dry filter paper on the conjunctiva. If the test is conducted carefully and excess fluid eliminated, it will detect a high percentage of those with aqueous-deficient dry eyes. In addition, many aqueous-deficient dry eyes, that would otherwise escape diagnosis, will be detected when reflex tearing due to the irritation of the dry strip is minimized or eliminated.

Author's procedure for the Schirmer test

1. Instil one drop of anaesthetic on both eyes, wait 2 minutes and instil a second drop
2. Wait 1 minute then depress the lower lid exposing the lower fornix. Roll a wick from soft absorbent tissue and place it at the junction between the middle and outer third of the lower eyelid into the inferior fornix to blot excess tears (simulating the placement of a Schirmer strip). The eye should be closed for 3–5 s, and then opened and the wick removed. Perform the procedure for the second eye, then repeat for both eyes
3. Place the Schirmer test paper at the junction between the middle and outer third of the lower eyelid, taking care not to irritate the cornea or conjunctiva. Repeat for the second eye
4. Instruct the patient to close both eyes gently, not to speak, and not to move the eyes in order to avoid contact between the test paper and the ocular surfaces. The head should be maintained in a horizontal position (an imaginary fixation target may be helpful)
5. After 5 minutes, remove the paper strip and record the wetted portion of the paper in mm as the final measurement.

References

Abdul-Fattah, A. M., Bhargava, H. N., Korb, D. R. *et al.* (1999) Quantitative in vitro comparison of fluorescein delivery to the eye via impregnated strip and volumetric techniques. ARVO Abstracts, *Invest. Ophthalmol. Vis. Sci.*, **40(4)**, S544.

Abelson, M. B. and Lamberts, D. W. (1983) Dry eye update. *Excerpta Medica (Amsterdam)*, 1–17.

Abelson, M. B. and Welch, D. (1994) How and why to treat dry eye. *Rev. Ophthalmol.*, **1(4)**, 58–59

Adams, A. D. (1979) The morphology of human conjunctival mucus. *Arch. Ophthalmol.*, **97**, 730–734.

Andres, S., Henriquez, A., Garcia, M. L. *et al.* (1987) Factors of the precorneal tear film break-up time (BUT) and tolerance of contact lenses. *Int. Cont. Lens Clin.*, **14(3)**, 103–107.

Awad, O. E., Goldstein, M. H. and Foulks, G. N. (1998) Inter- and intra-operator variability using the Advanced Nanoliter Osmometer™, Model 3000. ARVO Abstracts, *Invest. Ophthalmol. Vis. Sci.*, **39(4)**, 538.

Berliner, M. L. (1949) *Biomicroscopy of the Eye*. New York, Paul B. Hoeber, Vol. 1, p. 281.

Bron, A. J. (1997) The Doyne Lecture: Reflections on the Tears. *Eye*, **11**, 583–602.

Brown, W. C., Chen, T., Gouge, S. *et al.* (1989). *Guidance Documents for Class III Contact Lenses*. Silver Spring, Contact Lens Branch, Division of Ophthalmic Devices, Food and Drug Administration, pp. 72–86.

Caffery, B. E. and Josephson, J. E. (1991) Corneal staining after sequential instillations of fluorescein over 30 days. *Optom. Vis. Sci.*, **68(6),** 467–469.

CCLRU (1997) *Grading Scales*. University of New South Wales, Cornea and Contact Lens Research Unit.

Clinch, T. E., Benedetto, D. A., Felberg, N. T. and Laibson, P. R. (1983) Schirmer's test. *Arch. Ophthalmol.*, **101,** 1381–1386.

Craig, J. P. and Tomlinson, A. (1997) Importance of the lipid layer in human tear film stability and evaporation. *Optom. Vis. Sci.*, **74(1),** 8–13.

De Rötth, A. (1941) On the hypofunction of the lacrimal gland. *Am. J. Ophthalmol.*, **24,** 20–25.

Efron, N. (1998) Grading Scales for Contact Lens Complications. Supplement to *Contact Lens Complications*, Butterworth-Heinemann.

Egbert, P. R., Lauber, S. and Maurice, D. M. (1977) A simple conjunctival biopsy. *Am. J. Ophthalmol.*, **84,** 798–801.

Ehlers, N. (1965) The precorneal tear film. Biomicroscopical, histological and chemical investigations. *Acta Ophthalmol.*, **81(Suppl.),** 5–136.

Feenstra, R. P. G. and Tseng, S. C. G. (1992a) Comparison of fluorescein and rose bengal staining. *Ophthalmology,* **99(4),** 605–617.

Feenstra, R. P. G. and Tseng, S. C. G. (1992b) What is actually stained by rose bengal? *Arch. Opthalmol.*, **110,** 984–993.

Finnemore, V. M. and Korb, D. R. (submitted) The influence of fluorescein solution volume and elapsed time following instillation on break-up time measurements. Submitted for publication.

Foulks, G. N., Awad, O. E. and Goldstein, M. H. (1998) Tear osmometry: an evaluation of a new clinical instrument for keratoconjuncitivis sicca. ARVO Abstracts, *Invest. Ophthalmol. Vis. Sci.*, **39(4),** 645.

Fraunfelder, F. T. (1996) Drugs used primarily in ophthalmology. In *Drug-induced Ocular Side Effects* (eds F. T. Fraunfelder and J. A. Grove), Baltimore, William & Wilkins, p. 462.

Fullard, R. J. and Wilson, G. S. (1986) Investigation of sloughed corneal epithelial cells collected by non-invasive irrigation of the corneal surface. *Curr. Eye Res.*, **5(11),** 847–856.

Gasson, A. and Morris, J. (1998) *The Contact Lens Manual; A Practical Fitting Guide*, 2nd edn. Oxford, Butterworth-Heinemann, p. 382.

Gilbard, J. P. (1994) Dry eye disorders. In *Principles and Practice of Ophthalmology* (eds D. M. Albert and F. A. Jakobeic), Philadelphia,W. B. Saunders, pp. 257–276.

Gilbard, J. P. and Farris, R. L. (1979) Tear osmolarity and ocular surface disease in keratoconjunctivitis sicca. *Arch. Ophthalmol.*, **97,** 1642–1646.

Guillon, J. P. (1982) Tear film photography and contact lens wear. *J. Br. Cont. Lens Assoc.*, **5,** 84–87.

Guillon, J. P. (1986) Tear film structure and contact lenses. In *The Precorneal Tear Film in Health, Disease, and Contact Lens Wear* (ed. F. J. Holly), Lubbock, Dry Eye Institute, pp. 914–939.

Guillon, J. P. (1987) The tear film structure of the contact lens wearer. PhD thesis, The City University Department of Optometry and Visual Science.

Guillon, J. P. and Guillon, M. (1993) Tear film examination of the contact lens patient. *Optician*, **206(5421),** 21–29.

Guillon, M., Styles, E., Guillon, J. P. and Maïssa, C. (1997) Preocular tear film characteristics of non-wearers and soft contact lens wearers. *Optom. Vis. Sci.,* **74(5),** 273–279.

Hamano, H., Kawabe, H. and Mitsunaga, S. (1982) Even field bio-differential interference microscope. *Folia Ophthalmol. Japan,* **33,** 383–388.

Hamano, H., Hori, M., Kawabe, M. *et al.* (1979) Biodifferential interference microscopic observations on anterior segment of eye (First report: observations of precorneal tear film). *J. Japan Cont. Lens Soc.,* **21,** 229–231.

Henderson, J. W. and Prough, W. (1950) Influence of age and sex on flow of tears. *Arch. Ophthalmol.,* **43,** 224–231.

Holly, F. J. (1973) Formation and rupture of the tear film. *Exp. Eye Res.,* **15,** 515–525.

Holly, F. J. (1989) Diagnosis and treatment of dry eye syndrome. *Cont. Lens Spectrum,* **4(7),** 37.

Holly, F. J., Beebe, W. E. and Esquivel, E. D. (1986) Lacrimation kinetics in humans as determined by a novel technique. In *The Precorneal Tear Film in Health, Disease, and Contact Lens Wear* (ed. F. J. Holly), Lubbock, Dry Eye Institute, pp. 76–88.

Hom, M. M. and Shovlin, J. P. (1997) Dry eyes and contact lenses. In *Contact Lens Prescribing and Fitting* (ed. M. M. Hom), Boston, Butterworth-Heinemann, pp. 293–309.

Isreb, M. A., Greiner, J. V., Korb, D. R. *et al.* (in press) Correlation of lipid layer thickness measurements with fluorescein tear film breakup time and Schirmer test.

Jacobsen, L. T. H., Axel, T. E. and Hansen, B. U. (1989) Dry eyes or mouth: an epidemiologic study in Swedish adults, with special reference to primary Sjögren's syndrome. *J. Autoimmun.,* **2,** 521–527.

Jones, L. T. (1966) The lacrimal secretory system and its treatment. *Am. J. Ophthalmol.,* **62,** 47–60.

Jordan, A. and Baum, J. (1980) Basic tear flow, does it exist? *Ophthalmology,* **87,** 920–930.

Josephson, J. E. (1983) Appearance of the preocular tear film lipid layer. *Am. J. Optom. Physiol. Optics,* **60,** 883–887.

Josephson, J. E. and Caffery, B. E. (1992) Corneal staining characteristics after sequential instillations of fluorescein. *Optom. Vis. Sci.,* **69(7),** 570–573.

Kikkawa, Y. (1972) Normal corneal staining with fluorescein. *Exp. Eye Res.,* **14(1),** 13–20.

Kilp, H., Schmid, E., Kirchner, L. and Zipf-Pohl, A. (1986) Tear film observation by reflecting microscopy and differential interference contrast microscopy. In *The Precorneal Tear Film in Health, Disease, and Contact Lens Wear* (ed. F. J. Holly), Lubbock, Dry Eye Institute, pp. 564–569.

Klaassen, C. D. (1980) Principles of toxicology. In *The Pharmacological Basis of Therapeutics* (eds A. G. Gilman, L. S. Goodman and A. Gilman), New York, Macmillan, p. 1603.

Korb, D. R. (1994) Tear film – contact lens interactions. In *Lacrimal Gland, Tear Film and Dry Eye Syndromes* (ed. D. A. Sullivan), New York, Plenum Press, pp. 403–410.

Korb, D. R. and Greiner, J. V. (1994) Increase in tear film lipid layer thickness following treatment of meibomian gland dysfunction. In *Lacrimal Gland, Tear*

Film and Dry Eye Syndromes (ed. D. A. Sullivan), New York, Plenum Press, 293–298.

Korb, D. R. and Henriquez, A. S. (1980) Meibomian gland dysfunction and contact lens intolerance. *J. Am. Optom. Assoc.*, **51(3)**, 243–251.

Korb, D. R. and Herman, J. P. (1979) Corneal staining subsequent to sequential fluorescein instillations. *J. Am. Optom. Assoc.*, **50(3)**, 361–367.

Korb, D. R. and Korb, J. M. E. (1970) Corneal staining prior to contact lens wearing. *J. Am. Optom. Assoc.*, **41(3)**, 228–232.

Korb, D. R., Baron, D. F., Herman, J. P. *et al.* (1994) Tear film lipid layer thickness as a function of blinking. *Cornea*, **13(4)**, 354–359.

Korb, D. R., Greiner, J. V., Glonek, T. *et al.* (1996) Effect of periocular humidity on the tear film lipid layer. *Cornea*, **15(2)**, 129–134.

Korb, D. R., Finnemore, V. M., Herman, J. P. *et al.* (1999) A new method for the fluorescein break-up time test. ARVO Abstracts, *Invest. Ophthalmol. Vis. Sci.*, **40(4)**, S544.

Kurihashi, K. (1986) Diagnostic tests of lacrimal function using cotton threads. Abstracts 91 and 93. In the International Tear Film Program, 1984, and in *The Precorneal Tear Film in Health, Disease, and Contact Lens Wear* (ed. F. J. Holly), Lubbock, Dry Eye Institute, pp. 84–116.

Kurihashi, K., Yanagihara, N. and Honda, Y. (1977) A modified Schirmer test: the fine-thread method for measuring lacrimation. *J. Pediatr. Ophthalmol.*, **14**, 390–397.

Lamberts, D. W., Foster, S. C. and Perry, H. D. (1978) Schirmer's test after topical anesthesia and the tear meniscus height in normal eyes. *Arch. Ophthalmol.*, **97**, 1082–1085.

Larke, J. R. (1985) *The Eye in Contact Lens Wear*. London, Butterworth-Heinemann, pp. 92–93.

Larke, J. R. (1997) *The Eye in Contact Lens Wear*, 2nd edn. Oxford, Butterworth-Heinemann, pp. 32–33.

Lee, S. H. and Tseng, S. C. G. (1997) Rose bengal staining and cytologic characteristics associated with lipid tear deficiency. *Am. J. Ophthalmol.*, **124**, 736–750.

Lemp, M. A., Dohlman, C. H., Kuabara, T. *et al.* (1971) Dry eye secondary to mucus deficiency. *Trans. Am. Acad. Ophthalmol. Otolaryngol.*, **75**, 1223–1227.

Lemp, M. A. (1995) Report of the National Eye Institute/industry workshop on clinical trials in dry eyes. *CLAO. J.*, **21(4)**, 221–232.

Lemp, M. A. and Hamill, J. R. (1973) Factors affecting tear film break-up in normal eyes. *Arch. Ophthalmol.*, **89**, 103–105.

Lemp, M. A. and Mathers, W. D. (1986) The corneal surface in keratoconjunctivitis sicca. In *The Preocular Tear Film in Health, Disease, and Contact Lens Wear* (ed. F. J. Holly), Lubbock, Dry Eye Institute, pp. 840–846.

Lemp, M. A., Dohlman, Ch. and Holly, F. J. (1970) Corneal dessication despite normal tear volume. *Ann. Ophthalmol.*, **2**, 258–284.

Linton, R. G., Curnow, D. H. and Riley, W. J. (1961) The meibomian glands. An investigation into the secretion and some aspects of the physiology. *Br. J. Ophthalmol.*, **45**, 718–723.

Lohman, L. E., Rao, G. N., Tripathi, R. C. *et al.* (1982) In vivo specular microscopy of edematous human cornea epithelium with light and scanning electron microscopic correlation. *Ophthalmology*, **89(6)**, 621–629.

Lowther, G. E. (1993) Comparison of hydrogel contact lens patients with and without the symptoms of dryness. *Int. Cont. Lens Clin.*, **20,** 191.

Lowther, G. E. (1997) Examination of patients and predicting tear film-related problems with hydrogel lens wear. *Dryness, Tears, and Contact Lens Wear*, Boston, Butterworth-Heinemann, pp. 36–37.

Mackie, I. A. and Seal, D. V. (1981) The questionably dry eye. *Br. J. Ophthalmol.*, **65,** 2–9.

Madden, R. K., Paugh, J. R. and Wang, C. (1994) Comparative study of two non-invasive tear film stability techniques. *Curr. Eye Res.*, **13,** 263–270.

Marquardt, R., Stodmeister, R. and Christ, T. (1986) Modification of tear film break-up time test for increased reliability. In *The Precorneal Tear Film in Health, Disease, and Contact Lens Wear* (ed. F. J. Holly), Lubbock, Dry Eye Institute, pp. 57–63.

Mathers, W. D., Lane, J. A. and Zimmerman, M. B. (1996) Tear film changes associated with normal aging. *Cornea*, **15(3),** 229–234.

McCulley, J. P. and Sciallis, G. F. (1977) Meibomian keratoconjunctivitis. *Am. J. Ophthalmol.*, **84,** 788–793.

McDonald, J. E. (1968) Surface phenomena of tear films. *Trans. Am. Ophthalmol. Soc.*, **66,** 905–939.

McMonnies, C. W. and Ho, A. (1986) Marginal dry eye diagnosis: history versus biomicroscopy. In *The Precorneal Tear Film in Health, Disease and Contact Lens Wear* (ed. F. J. Holly), Lubbock, Dry Eye Institute, pp. 32–40.

McMonnies, C. W. and Ho, A. (1987) Patient history in screening for dry eye conditions. *J. Am. Optom. Assoc.*, **58,** 296.

McMonnies, C., Ho, A. and Wakefield, D. (1998) Optimum dry eye classification using questionnaire responses. In *Lacrimal Gland, Tear Film and Dry Eye Syndromes 2* (ed. D. A. Sullivan), New York, Plenum Press, pp. 835–838.

Mengher, L. S., Bron, A. J., Tonge, S. R. and Gilbert, D. J. (1985a) A non-invasive instrument for clinical assessment of the precorneal tear film stability. *Curr. Eye Res.*, **4,** 1–7.

Mengher, L. S., Bron, A. J., Tonge, S. R. and Gilbert, D. J. (1985b) Effect of fluorescein instillation on the precorneal tear film stability. *Curr. Eye Res.*, **4(1),** 9–12.

Mengher, L. S., Bron, A. J., Tonge, S. R. and Gilbert, D. J. (1986) Non-invasive assessment of tear film stability. In *The Precorneal Tear Film in Health, Disease, and Contact Lens Wear* (ed. F. J. Holly), Lubbock, Dry Eye Institute, pp. 64–75.

Merrill, D. L., Fleming, T. C. and Girard, L. J. (1960) The effects of physiologic balanced salt solution and normal saline on intraocular and extraocular tissues. *Am. J. Ophthalmol.*, **49,** 895.

Mishima, S., Gasset, A., Klyce, S. D. and Baum, J. L. (1966) Determination of tear volume and tear flow. *Invest. Ophthalmol.*, **5,** 264–276.

Murube, J. (1992) History of the dry eye. In *The Dry Eye. A Comprehensive Guide* (eds M. A. Lemp and R. Marquardt), Berlin, Springer-Verlag, p. 12.

Nelson, J. D. (1982) Ocular surface impressions using cellulose acetate filter material. Ocular pemphigoid. *Surv. Ophthal.*, **27(1),** 67–69.

Nelson, J. D. (1994) Diagnosis of keratoconjunctivitis sicca. *Int. Ophthalmol. Clin.*, **34,** 37–56.

Norn, M. S. (1960) Cytology of the conjunctival fluid. *Acta Ophthalmol. (Kbh)*, **59(Suppl.)**, 1–152.

Norn, M. S. (1969) Dessication of the precorneal tear film. I. Corneal wetting time. *Acta Ophthalmol.*, **47**, 865–880.

Norn, M. S. (1970) Micropunctate fluorescein vital staining of the cornea. *Acta Ophthalmol.*, **48**, 108–118.

Norn, M. S. (1972) Vital staining of cornea and conjunctiva. *Acta Ophthalmol.*, **50**, 286–294.

Norn, M. S. (1973) Lissamine green. Vital staining of cornea and conjunctiva. *Acta Ophthalmol.*, **51(4)**, 483–491.

Norn, M. S. (1974) Examination after vital staining. In *External Eye. Methods of Examination*. Copenhagen, Scriptor, pp. 51–72.

Norn, M. S. (1979) Semiquantitative interference study of fatty layer of precorneal film. *Acta Ophthalmol.*, **57**, 766–774.

Norn, M. S. (1992) Diagnosis of dry eye. In *The Dry Eye. A Comprehensive Guide* (eds M. A. Lemp and R. Marquardt), Berlin, Springer-Verlag, pp. 165–169.

Patel, S., Murray, D., McKenzie, A. *et al.* (1985) Effects of fluorescein on tear break-up time and on tear thinning time. *Am. J. Optom. Physiol. Opt.*, **62(3)**, 188–190.

Pflugfelder, S. C. (1996) Differential diagnosis of dry eye conditions. *Adv. Dent. Res.*, **10(1)**, 9–12.

Pflugfelder, S. C., Tseng, S. C., Sanabria, O. *et al.* (1998) Evaluation of subjective assessments and objective diagnostic tests for diagnosing tear-film disorders known to cause ocular irritation. *Cornea*, **17(1)**, 38–56.

Rengstorff, R. H. (1974) The precorneal tear film: break-up time and location in normal subjects. *Am. J. Optom. Physiol. Optics*, **51**, 765–769.

Rolando, M., Macri, A., Carlandrea, T. and Calabria, G. (1998) Use of a questionnaire for the diagnosis of tear film-related ocular surface disease. In *Lacrimal Gland, Tear Film and Dry Eye Syndromes 2* (ed. D. A. Sullivan), New York, Plenum Press, pp. 822–825.

Schein, O. D., Munoz, B. and Tielsch, J. M. (1996) Estimating the prevalence of dry eye among elderly Americans: SEE Project. ARVO Abstracts, *Invest. Ophthalmol. Vis. Sci.*, **37**, S636.

Snyder, C. and Paugh, J. R. (1998) Rose bengal dye concentration and volume delivered via dye-impregnated paper strips. *Optom. Vis. Sci.*, **75(5)**, 339–341.

Strickland, R. W., Tesar, J. T. and Beene, B. H. (1987) The frequency of sicca syndrome in an elderly population. *J. Rheumatol.*, **14**, 766–771.

Tearscope (1997) *Tearscope Plus Clinical Hand Book and Tearscope Plus Instructions*. Windsor, Keeler Ltd, Windsor, Berkshire; Keeler Insts Inc., Broomall, PA.

Thomas, M. L., Szeto, V. R., Gan, C. M. and Polse, K. A. (1997) Sequential staining: the effects of sodium fluorescein, osmolarity, and pH on human corneal epithelium. *Optom. Vis. Sci.*, **74(4)**, 207–210.

Tomlinson, A. (1992) Contact lens-induced dry eye. In *Complications of Contact Lens Wear* (ed. A. Tomlinson), St Louis, Mosby, pp. 195–218.

Tonge, S. R., Hunsaker, J. and Holly, F. J. (1991) Non-invasive assessment of tear film break-up time in a group of normal subjects – implications for contact lens wear. *J. Br. Cont. Lens Assoc.*, **14**, 201–205.

Tseng, S. C. G. (1994) Evaluation of the ocular surface in dry eye conditions. *Int. Ophthal. Clin.*, **34(1)**, 57–69.

van Bijsterveld, O. P. (1969) Diagnostic tests in the sicca syndrome. *Arch. Ophthalmol.*, **82**, 10–14.

Vanley, G. T., Leopold, I. H. and Gregg, T. H. (1977) Interpretation of tear film break-up. *Arch. Ophthalmol.*, **95**, 445–448.

Wilson, G., Ren, H. and Laurent, J. (1995) Corneal epithelial fluorescein staining. *J. Am. Optom. Assoc.*, **66(7)**, 435–441.

Wolff, E. (1946) The muco-cutaneous junction of the lid margin and the distribution of the tear fluid. *Trans. Ophthalmol. Soc. UK*, **66**, 291–308.

Yokoi, N., Takehisa, Y. and Kinoshita, S. (1996) Correlation of tear lipid layer interference patterns with the diagnosis and severity of dry eye. *Am. J. Ophthalmol.*, **122**, 818–824.

Zengin, N., Tol, H., Gunduz, K. *et al.* (1995) Meibomian gland dysfunction and tear film abnormalities in rosacea. *Cornea*, **14**, 144–146.

Index